Shadow Yoga
Chaya Yoga

Shadow Yoga
Chaya Yoga

The Principles of Hatha Yoga

Shandor Remete

North Atlantic Books
Berkeley, California

Published by
North Atlantic Books
P.O. Box 12327
Berkeley, California 94712

Cover design by Suzanne Albertson
Book design by Detour Design
Edited by John Evans
Illustrated by Joey Huynh
Calligraphy by Nakamura Taisaburo Sensei
Printed in the United States of America

Shadow Yoga, Chaya Yoga: The Principles of Hatha Yoga is sponsored by the Society for the Study of Native Arts and Sciences, a nonprofit educational corporation whose goals are to develop an educational and cross-cultural perspective linking various scientific, social, and artistic fields; to nurture a holistic view of arts, sciences, humanities, and healing; and to publish and distribute literature on the relationship of mind, body, and nature.

North Atlantic Books' publications are available through most bookstores. For further information, call 800-733-3000 or visit our Web site at www.northatlanticbooks.com.

Library of Congress Cataloging-in-Publication Data
Remete, Shandor, 1948–
    Shadow yoga, Chaya yoga : the principles of Hatha yoga / Shandor Remete.
        p. cm.
    Includes bibliographical references and index.
        Summary: "Shadow Yoga is an elegant, concise treatise on the hidden roots of yoga. Beautiful drawings and photographs illustrate the subtle concepts and Sanskrit terminology underpinning the poses"—Provided by publisher.
    ISBN 978-1-55643-876-9
    1. Yoga. I. Title.
    B132.Y6R433 2009
    181'.45—dc22

                                    2009036822

2 3 4 5 6 7 8 9 UNITED 14 13 12 11 10

Dedicated to Ms. Emma Balnaves, without whom this world of material appearances would seem like an eternal prison of suffering.

And to my children Emeshe, Arikan, Noemi, and Atreya, to whom my absence has caused an excess of pain, yet I carry them deep in my heart. May God forgive me.

Contents

Preface

I would like to begin by paying my respects to all the people who have been instrumental in the cultivation of the intelligence that flows through me. This intelligence guides me along the yogic path like a flaming torch, dispelling the darkness of ignorance. Beyond all others, I bow to Lord Shiva, the great God of Yogis and Wanderers on the path.

I was introduced to the practice of yoga at the young age of six by my father. Through his example I learned all the basic asanas, *kriyas,* and *bandhas.* His guidance was patient and persistent yet unimposed. Later, I studied for two decades under the firm hand and watchful eye of yoga master B. K. S. Iyengar of Pune, India.

During this time, I also had the good fortune to receive some of the early writings of Sri T. Krishnamacharya of Madras (present-day Chennai). Among these, one short work has influenced me profoundly: *Salutations to the Teacher and the Eternal One.* It has been this book more than any other that has helped me to decipher and understand the ancient hatha yogic texts in their fullness. And it is this growing understanding that has determined my course over time.

This little book you are now holding, *Shadow Yoga,* is the culmination of what I have studied, read, and practiced thus far. Its fourteen chapters have been woven together from threads drawn from the classical hatha yoga texts, that the knowledge may become more accessible to the sincere seeker. There is nothing in this book that I have not tested and put to use over many years of training, day and night.

During that time I have explored both the well-known and the lesser-known styles of present-day yoga, their advantages as well as their disadvantages. I have also studied other disciplines: martial arts and the ancient Kathakali and Bharatanatyam dance forms of southern India. What has become apparent to me is that there is a common basis in the preparatory forms of all of these disciplines.

Preparatory forms are essential for the learning of and the unfolding of the energetic principles of the yoga practice. Although they have been (and are still) utilized in the afore-mentioned disciplines over the ages, they are no longer found or known about in the popular styles of modern-day yoga. This lack of basic preparatory activity leaves the beginner wide open to confusion, injury, and empty promises.

Throughout the ages, the cultivation of power has always been achieved through very simple and uncomplicated movements. The prelude forms of the Shadow School of yoga are not a new invention but a resurrection of what is an age-old method of preparing the body, mind, and spirit.

The theoretical information contained within this book is therefore offered to nourish the seeds of the divine energy that is hidden deep within the human form, that it may unfold.

Shandor Remete
Adelaide, Australia, 2006

How to Use This Book

The prelude sequences illustrated in this book can be memorized and then practiced using the understanding gained from reading the text. This process of *bahiranga sadhana* will be enhanced by careful observation of the Shadow Yoga DVDs. The practice of *yogasanas*, however, cannot be learned from books or audiovisual tools alone. The internal processes, *antaranga sadhana* of *yogasanas*, *pranayamas*, *kriyas*, *bandhas*, and *mudras* must be learned with the guidance of a teacher well-versed in this style so that these practices can be introduced and adapted according to the needs of the individual.

The theoretical information contained in this book is intended to evoke an understanding of universal principles that the mind can rest upon during practice. Detailed technical information, on the other hand, will pollute the mind and prevent absorption in the practice. The role of the teacher is to introduce technical points only when they are called for in order that the individual student can relate appropriately to the activity. As the practitioner matures and action is carried out in accordance with universal principles the necessary techniques hidden within the forms and movements will spontaneously reveal themselves. If the student practices the prelude forms diligently, with correct rhythm and attention, they will begin to experience this process of realization for themselves.

The *mudras* spoken of within this text should not be attempted. They relate to *paramantaranga sadhana* and are included here only to indicate the direction in which advanced practice should move. Many suggestions are contained in them that only time and diligent practice will reveal. In the later stages only a few asanas are required for the spiritual unfolding of the individual. In the early stages

milder forms of these asanas are learned from an experienced teacher as the appropriate preludes are mastered.

Only an outline of the basic asanas, *kriyas, bandhas,
pranayamas, mudras,* and *pratyahara* is given in this book
since all these practices should be learned directly under
the guidance of an experienced teacher who is well-versed
in all aspects of the art, craft, and science of yoga.

Part 1
Knowledge

1
Shadow Yoga

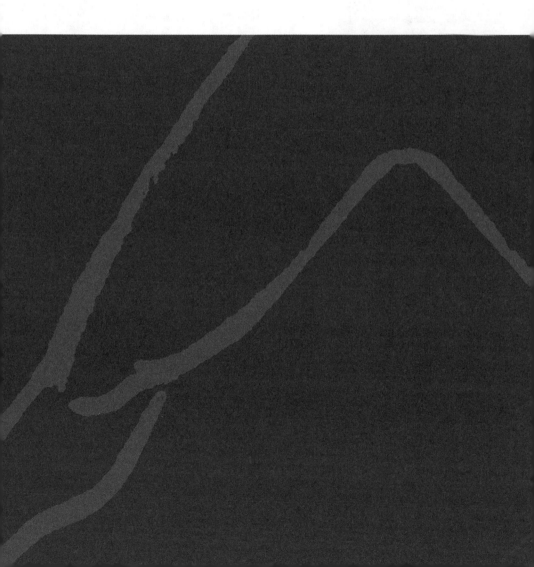

Before opening a discussion on Shadow Yoga it is important to grasp the meaning hidden behind the term *yoga* itself. Yoga is a spiritual system that deals practically with the process of enlightenment. The final goal is to differentiate the soul from everything that is not the soul. The method of yoga teaches the individual to discriminate, or to see the differences between these two things.

This process involves the skillful reduction of fixed patterns within the individual that obstruct or distort perception of reality and so create confusion. If we are constantly mindful of this end goal, to distinguish the soul from everything that is not the soul, we will always be able to choose the correct means for making the next step toward a successful completion of the yogic journey.

In the third verse of the *Hatha Yoga Pradipika,* Svatmarama Yogendra states, "For those who are deluded by the multiplicity of views and are ignorant of Raja Yoga, Svatmarama compassionately puts forth the lesson of *Hatha Pradipika.*" Reflection on the hidden meaning of this verse reveals that what is being offered here is a form of skillful means. This consists of the necessary equipment, instructions for its use, and a description of what is to be attained from that use. Hatha yoga is the equipment; *avadhuta yoga* (asceticism) is the skillful use of the equipment, while *raja yoga* is the fruit obtained from that use. These three together constitute *maha yoga.* Unless these three are viewed as parts of one whole they lose their meaning.

Asana, *kriya, pranayama, mudra, yantra, mantra,* and *laya* are all types of equipment. The right tool applied at the appropriate time in a skillful manner is *hatha-avadhuta yoga,* which is the manifestation of the *yamas* (restraints) and *niyamas* (observances). Skillful activity is unobstructed, nonharmful behavior, which brings about the merging of the two opposing energies of the sun *(ha)* and moon *(tha).*

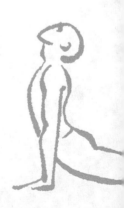

This is *raja yoga* or *siddha* (attained) *yoga*. The moon is the shadow body of the sun, yet it reflects the life-supporting light of this star. Shadow Yoga *(chaya yoga)* is a synonym for hatha yoga that emphasizes this truth.

Hatha-avadhuta yoga is the beginning of the path, while *raja yoga* or *siddha yoga* is the goal. When this is achieved, the individual no longer practices but lives according to the one universal Truth that binds all. The noose or reins *(pasha)* represents the body of laws that governs the various elements of matter and living beings in creation. *Pashupati* is the shining herdsman who, through *pati* (mastery), has risen above *pashu* (animalistic existence).

The Shadow School is built upon these principles. By investigating the shadow and its source we come to light. Since yoga is the reversal of the manifestation of life, one must start with the shadows. By coming to understand them, we can dissolve them. When the light of the sun and moon comes into contact with objects, shadows are created. According to one of the forefathers of hatha yoga, Allama Prabhudeva, "The appearance of this body is nothing but layers of frozen shadows."

These shadows are seven in number: the shadow of joy, the shadow of the intellect, the shadow of the mundane mind, the power principle, the gross structure, the luster of the skin, and the shadow on the ground. Each shadow is a blockage of light. By considering the list of shadows given here one can see how different people are stuck on different planes. Some are joy hunters, some are power mongers, while others are intellectuals, and so on. There is nothing wrong with any of these kinds of behavior, but by themselves they lead nowhere. However, if these shadows are correctly investigated with an open mind, then they can fuel the journey to enlightenment.

The *Siva Svarodaya*, an ancient *tantrika* text on the life breath *(svara)*, contains a short chapter entitled "Yoga of the Shadow Man." It describes how to observe one's own shadow and recognize the many symptoms hidden within it. Verse 382 states: "If the shadow does not have any head the man will die within a period of one month, if it does not have any thigh he will die within eight days ..."

In *Charaka Samhita*, section *Indriya Sthana*, chapter 7, the following interpretation of the shadow and luster is given: "If there is any deformity observed in body parts in the shadow of the person in moonlight, sunlight, the light of a lamp, water or mirror he should be considered a ghost." These references reveal how the shadows can be used as diagnostic tools to ascertain where we are at any given moment. It should be borne in mind, however, that the shadows hidden in the deeper recesses require correspondingly much closer observation.

The process of enlightenment is a dynamic evolving activity, and not a fixed state of attachment, as many conceive it to be. The practice of yoga requires an open, fluid, and sensitive mind, which should not be confused with an emotional mind. Although many present-day styles describe themselves as both fluid and flowing, the focusing on any one quality or attribute conceals a very lack of openness and fluidity. Whether it be flowing style, soft style, power-based or alignment-oriented, the very focus demonstrates that the mind is infatuated with one aspect of the practice. This leads to excessive use of techniques or movements or points of adjustment that results in an unnecessary waste of time and energy. The complex and attractive appearance of such styles conceals a lack of roots.

Hatha yoga is a system of self-cultivation by which the individual frees himself from the burden of the world and its bondage.

This cannot be achieved through superficial work. One must begin at the root and grow slowly, grow with patience, and grow through persistence. Boredom is overcome by paying keen attention to the activity.

The early texts on hatha yoga all agree on the nine most important asanas, namely *bhekasana, bhujangasana, mandukasana, kurmasana, mayurasana, bhadrasana, siddhasana, baddha padmasana,* and *kukkutasana.* These nine asanas are the seeds for all the innumerable possibilities that are available to any individual who possesses the necessary wisdom to work with those seeds.

Every beginner is faced with a set formula to learn which, by its very nature, carries the inherent danger of attachment. In yoga these formulas, or preludes, as I term them, are vital for the proper cultivation of the key asanas. The individual works with the preludes and the key asanas in three stages of mild, medium, and intense. To progress in this way one must understand the rhythm of prelude, *asana-vinyasa* (progressive use of asana), and conclusion, as well as the principle of counter posing. Every asana has its counter pose and unless this is known the individual will be confronted by unnecessary setbacks or injuries.

The prelude forms consist of warrior and sun forms. The warrior forms are circular and spiral, while the sun forms are linear. These forms are carried out in a flowing manner and they should be learned first and practiced daily for three to seven years before beginning the *asana-vinyasa.* The warrior forms free the peripheral body from its tensions and energetic obstructions, while the sun forms ignite the central power system.

Only when the preludes have been mastered should the work on the key asanas begin. The problem that beginners encounter today is the premature exposure to difficult asanas. The struggles that result excite their minds but blind them to the natural order of progression in the asanas. Failing to build a foundation, they fall short of their goal. Their impatience is born of ignorance of the simplicity of the system.

All the asanas fall into one of five categories: bending forward, bending to the side, bending backward, twisting, and balancing. These five actions can be done standing, sitting, lying face down, face up, on one's side, or inverted. These five bodily positions correspond to the *pancha mukhas* (five faces) of Lord Shiva.

The same insight applies to martial arts and is contained in the work of Japan's most famous swordsman, Miyamoto Musashi, *The Book of Five Rings*. He criticizes other sword schools for flowery and unnecessary techniques that are useless in combat, stating, "There are only five ways to cut a person down, the vertical downward cut, the horizontal cut, the diagonal up and diagonal down cuts and the thrust." Everything else, he says, is a variation of these five possibilities according to the needs of a given situation.

Most people today are too stiff and unfit for even the so-called beginner asanas like *janu sirsasana* or *urdhva dhanurasana*, never mind the twists, balances, and side bends. By prematurely attempting these positions beginner students end up overusing their arms to compensate for stiff hips or shoulders to pull or push the body into position. Overuse of the arms in this way causes the subtle body (the power structure) to weaken and rupture. This type of misguided behavior can result in weakening of the throat, heart, navel, perineal, and rectal regions, triggering the enlargement of the liver and spleen and malfunctions of the pancreas. These are the dangers that the beginner unknowingly confronts.

Simple asanas that are often overlooked yield many benefits, when properly utilized. For example, *swastikasana* (sun
wheel) demands a direct action from the ankles while indirectly affecting all the other joints, including the spine. It is
little understood that the flexibility of the whole body can
be achieved through the proper manipulation of the ankles,
wrists, and neck. When these five regions are flexible the
entire system softens and gains elasticity.

Mandukasana (the seated frog), another basic seat, together
with its variations, affects the hips and the shoulders
directly, and all the other areas indirectly. It is the bridge
between preparatory work and forward and backward
bends. As its name suggests, *mandukasana* mirrors the rest-
ing position in which many members of the frog family
hibernate. There is an indication here that the removal of
stiffness in the hips and shoulders gained in this asana
improves respiration.

The hatha yoga system is designed to bring about a cessation of respiration without aggression. This short reflection
on these two postures indicates how their proper use pre-
pares the body in many ways for the practice of asana,
bandha, kriya, pranayama, mudra, and *laya.*

The above nine key positions have their primary, intermediate, and advanced levels which should all be learned before
one discards the fixed forms and enters the practice of
freestyle. The practice of the fixed forms without their preludes and conclusions will result in few, if any, benefits. Only
when these nine most important asanas have been mastered is the beginner ready for the hatha yogic journey
proper. The practice of yoga will fail due to an excess of one
or more of the following: food, exertion, talking, austerity,
public contact, and greed.

The essence of the Shadow School teachings is contained in the compound noun *kaya-sama-sthana-ghati-kriya*. *Kaya* refers to the body, *sama* means "even" or "equal," *sthana* refers to bodily placement or a stance, *ghati* is a standard unit of time of twenty-four minutes, and *kriya* means "process." The full compound translates as "a process undergone through a sequence of equalizing movements over a period of twenty-four minutes." The term *ghati* is often used in the texts to refer to the duration of different forms of practice and is defined as the length of time it takes for the energy to circulate once around the body. When the implications of *kaya-sama-sthana-ghati-kriya* are properly understood, the six possible causes of failure will be overcome.

A complete session of yogic practice consists of asana, *kriya, pranayama, mudra,* and *laya* (absorption). Asana itself is made up of the three steps of prelude, chosen *asana-vinyasa,* and conclusion. As *ghati* in the above compound suggests, any unit of practice should be carried out within twenty-four minutes (one *ghati*) since it takes this much time for the energy to complete a full cycle around the body. According to the texts, the practice is fulfilled when the *prana* is contained within the body and is exercised continuously for five *ghatika* (two hours).

Kaya-sama-sthana-ghati-kriya also conveys the idea of a many-faceted, organic, rhythmic development through the complete practice. The three phases of each form (prelude, *asana-vinyasa,* and conclusion) together with *kriya, pranayama, bandha,* and *mudra* equip the practitioner with the necessary responsiveness to the rhythmic qualities of *prana* for the state of *laya* (absorption), the desired goal of all yogic activities. The rhythmic changes experienced in the different activities neutralize the buildup of greed, the root cause of excessive and obsessive behavior, which so often results in failure, not only in yoga but also in other areas of life.

If the mind remains open and fluid without wavering or losing the direction of action, a well-planned yoga session will reflect the saying that all motion ends in stillness while stillness ends in motion.

2
Mitahara: The Controlled Intake of Pure Foods

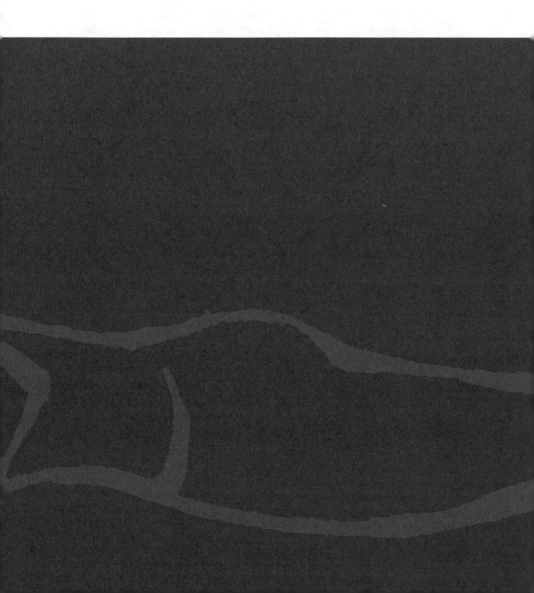

At the beginning of every new subject in ancient Indian texts, the word *atha* appears. Most readers pass over this single word without realizing its great significance. It indicates that something else, something unstated should have taken place before this new subject is approached. Without the proper application of the preceding information a person who undertakes the next step will stumble. This conveys a warning that one should thoroughly investigate the required preliminaries before engaging in experimentation.

Bearing this in mind, the beginner should tread with caution when acquiring theoretical knowledge. They should not forget that they are dealing with the practical science of yoga. Theoretical information should never be imposed upon the practice; instead it should be used as a method for observing one's behavior. It must not interfere with the natural movements of the limbs and the pranic force. It provides the beginner with a map of the energetic sites and pathways, and serves as a device by which one can check one's personal growth in the practices of asana, *kriya, bandha, pranayama, mudra,* and *laya.*

Theoretical information should be digested until it feels as if the information has sprung forth and grown from within one's own self. Practice and theory will then be one inseparable living knowledge manifesting as wisdom and action at all times. This is the required state of mind for the opening of the gate to the path of yoga. Until this point is reached the practice will exist as a reality separate from oneself. Yoga is the art of merging all differing forces into one. The beginner must strive without tiring until their continuous efforts bring forth the key that unlocks their inner power. Before information about energetic locations and circuits can be utilized it is important to reflect upon dietary habits, and to modify them appropriately. This helps to overcome greed-related abuse. The *Chandogya*

Upanishad gives a concise analysis of the breakdown of food in the human system:

> The gross part of solids becomes feces; the middle part becomes flesh, while the subtle becomes mind.
>   The gross part of fluid becomes urine, the middle part blood and the subtle part breath.
>   The gross part of fire (digestive process) becomes bone, the middle part becomes marrow and the fine part becomes speech.

From this, one can see that by controlling the intake of solids one gains control over the physical body and the mind. From control over solids we gain control indirectly over the fluids, blood, and breath. It is at the blood level that the practice of yoga begins. A polluted bloodstream results in poor respiration. The proper practice of asana and *pranayama* automatically reduces the quantity of feces and urine. This instantly increases the inner heat as well as the quality of bone and marrow.

An undisciplined mind is responsible for the pollution of blood and a reduction in the quality of the inner light. Before one attempts the practice of yoga one should investigate one's dietary habits and learn to curb them to a degree. The diet eventually should be fully vegetarian and restricted to a few foods that are agreeable to the individual.

The hatha yogic texts suggest the use of three grains—rice, barley, and wheat; some leafy and root vegetables with mild spices; and sweets like honey, candy sugar, and maple syrup. Each individual should experiment with their food until they discover what is easily digestible for them, and use only those foods.

The controlled intake of these chosen foods should not be imposed, but introduced gradually over a period of time. It should be pleasing for the body as a whole and not just the palate. Salty, sour, and excessively bitter foods should be avoided. Sweet, astringent, and slightly pungent spices like black pepper, cloves, ginger, cinnamon, and cardamom can be used freely.

By controlling the palate one gains control over the body and the mind, the blood is cleaned, the breath becomes powerful, and one gains good bones, marrow, and gentle speech.

3
The Planets and Signs of the Zodiac and Their Influence on the Human System

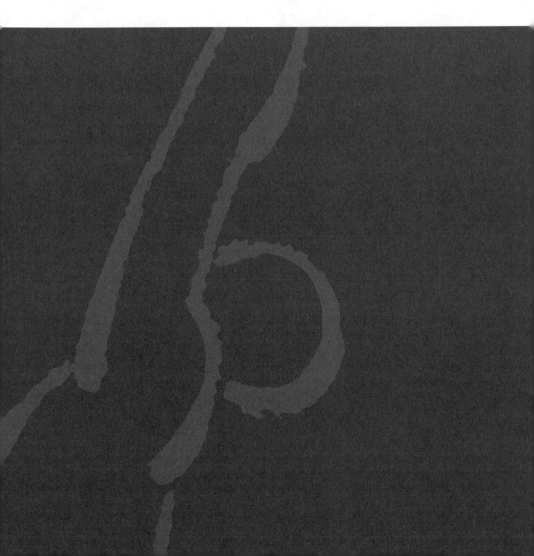

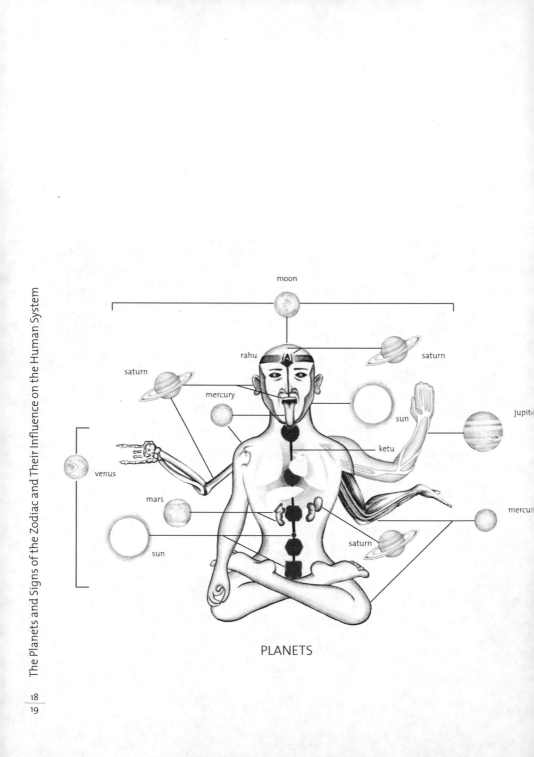

moon

rahu

saturn

mercury

saturn

sun

ketu

jupit

venus

mars

mercu

sun

saturn

PLANETS

The universe and the human being are related as a macrocosm is to a microcosm. The human being is constituted from light particles derived from the sun, the moon, the planets of the solar system, and the different star formations of the zodiac. Because of this, it is important to know which heavenly bodies rule the various bodily parts and how they exert influence upon them. While these influences are sometimes benevolent, occasionally they also exert a malevolent influence. One should become well acquainted with all of these relationships so that one can utilize good influences for one's growth and recognize when not to force things while negative influences are at work.

The sun presides over the area of the navel and the face, and controls the subtle body. The moon governs the top of the brain and controls the entire physical body. Mars manages the gall bladder and kidneys. Mercury governs the tongue, arms, and legs, as well as the nerves, ligaments, sinews, tendons, and other soft tissues. Jupiter is in charge of the blood, blood vessels, and skin. Venus controls all the organs between the throat and the perineal floor, including the genitals. Saturn oversees the third eye, the ears, the teeth, and all the bones and joints, as well as the spleen and the brain. Rahu, the north node of the moon, controls the midsection of the brain from the middle of the forehead through to the whorl of the hair, while Ketu, the south node of the moon, regulates the spinal cord.

The sun, Mars, and Saturn are malefic by nature, while the other signs are benevolent and influenced by the moon. The twelve signs of the zodiac are divided equally between the sun and the moon.

The sun signs and the bodily parts they affect are: Aries on the neck and throat; Gemini on the arms, hands, and fingers; Leo on the heart and stomach; Libra on the kidneys;

Sagittarius on the hips; and Aquarius on the thighs and shins. As the sun is in charge of the subtle body, it is through these body parts and organs that the subtle body is brought into action during the different yogic practices. The subtle body and its related organs can be controlled through the channel of the right nostril *(pingala nadi)*.

The moon signs and the bodily parts they influence are: Taurus on the shoulders and shoulder blades; Cancer on the rib cage; Virgo on the intestines; Scorpio on the genitals; Capricorn on the knees; and Pisces on the feet. As the moon is in charge of these body parts and organs, they can be controlled through the channel of the left nostril *(ida nadi)*.

This information is of great importance to the yoga practitioner since it enables modification of the practice according to favorable and unfavorable conditions. Injuries and many illnesses can be avoided through understanding these influences. Since yoga is the science of harmony, and we are only manifestations of the heavenly bodies, one should understand their areas of influence on our bodies. It is only in this way that one can neutralize the effects of the planets. This provides one of the keys to knowing what to do, when to do it, how to do it, and how much of it to do.

4
The Energetic Circuits of the Microcosmic Systems and Their Locations

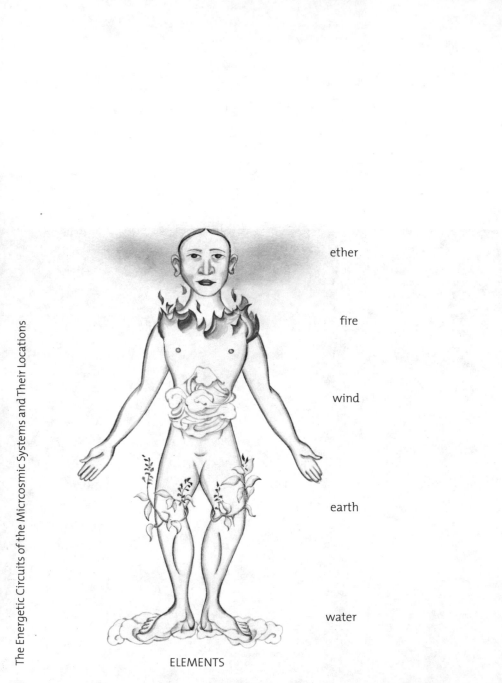

ether

fire

wind

earth

water

ELEMENTS

Human beings are the product of the five basic elements of sky (ether), wind, fire, water, and earth. These are the constituent materials of the complex energetic systems of both the macrocosmic body of the universe and the microcosmic body of the individual.

According to the yoga texts, the human form is made up of three distinct bodies, five traps (encasements or sheaths), 108 vital junctions (points), seven energy centers, ten winds, and 72,000 energetic flows or channels. Of these channels, thirteen are important. Of those thirteen, three are of great importance. And of those three, one is of supreme importance.

There are nine gates in the human body through which energy can be conserved or dissipated. There are five organs of perception (ears, skin, eyes, tongue, and nose), and their related qualities (sound, touch, sight, taste, and smell), and five organs of action (mouth, hands, feet, genitals, and anus), all of which correspond to the five elements.

Among the organs of perception, the tongue plays a central role in conducting energy between the peripheral and central channels. It consequently has a major influence on the physiological functions of the body.

When these many energy systems work harmoniously there is synergy; they act together as a single unit. But when any one part malfunctions the whole system begins to break down. All yoga practitioners should be well-informed about the functioning of this whole system because this is the only trustworthy theoretical foundation for a well-balanced practice. Without knowledge of the energetic systems one is likely to waste many years of effort and good intentions, scratching in the dark.

The correct movement of the limbs triggers all of these systems. The limbs can be moved naturally in a harmonious manner, or unnaturally and without harmony. This is why it is vital to start with simple and uncomplicated movements that allow the individual to observe and discover the natural and inherent actions of the limbs. Forcing movement leads to distortion and disharmony. The pranic force can only be awakened through harmonious rhythmic activity, and unless one is aware of the energetic circuits and locations one will not know how to look for this. Ether is located in the forehead, its related organ of sense is the ears, and the organ of action is the mouth (tongue). Wind is located at the base of the navel, it correlates to the sense organ of the skin, and the hands are its organs of action. Fire is located in the shoulders, and its organs of sense are the eyes, the feet its organs of action. Water is located in the feet, the organ of sense is the tongue, and the organs of action are the genitals. Earth is located in the knees, the organ of sense is the nose, and the anus is the organ of action.

Ether is responsible for sound, wind for touch, fire for form, water for taste, and earth for scent. The earth's color is yellow, water's is white, fire is red, and the color related to air is black, while ether is multicolored. Each element has a symbol: the earth a square, water a crescent moon, fire a triangle, wind a circle, and ether a point.

Earth is located in the center, water flows downwards, fire burns upwards, wind blows to the sides, while ether is perceived at every intersection of the other elements. The corresponding flavors are: earth is bland, water is astringent, fire is pungent, air is acidic, ether is bitter. Each element exerts an action: earth engenders stability; water creates movement; cruel acts belong to fire; killing and cursing belong to the wind; and the ether is good for meditative activities only. Within each hour of the day, earth dominates for twenty minutes, water for sixteen minutes, fire for twelve minutes, wind for eight minutes, and ether for four minutes. The sequence of dominance is wind first, then fire, water, earth, and finally ether.

Knowledge of the five elements and what they correspond to is of great importance to yoga practitioners. It helps to determine the choice and the appropriate rhythm of practice. To ensure good results, the practice of asana should always start when either earth or water is ruling. If the practice of asana is started when either wind, fire, or ether is ruling, one faces the strong possibility of injuries and disappointing setbacks.

It is also important to be aware of the appropriate times of the day that are conducive to yoga practices in order to avoid impediments to success. These times are before sunrise, at midday, before sunset, and before midnight. Out of these, dawn and dusk are most suitable for beginners. For particularly stiff people, dusk is more appropriate than dawn, since the body has warmed up during the activities of the day and the practice will require less effort. The most important thing is to use this information to maximize results while minimizing the expenditure of energy. The three bodies within the human system are the causal, *karana sharira,* the subtle, *sukshma sharira* and the gross, *sthula sharira.* The causal body is the seat and origin of the individual soul *(jiva).* Without the causal body, no manifestation of life is possible. The subtle body is the outpouring of the causal body in the form of life force *(prana).* The subtle body is responsible for all life functions within the gross structure of the physical form (the *sthula sharira*).

According to the texts of both yoga and Ayurveda, these three bodies also include a number of *koshas. Kosha* is usually translated as "sheath" or "encasement," but a better translation is "entrapment" or "trap," since this conveys the important nuance of limitation or bondage.

Yoga texts list five of these traps, while Ayurveda texts list seven. The *koshas* interweave the three bodies, and are responsible for the integration of the different life functions of the individual. The *koshas* are expressions of the pranic force. They are dissolved back into their original source through the transformative processes stimulated by yogic practices.

Annamaya kosha is the trap of food, *pranamaya kosha* is the trap of power, *manomaya kosha* is the trap of the processing mind, *vijnanamaya kosha* is the trap of the intuitive intellect, and *anandamaya kosha* is the trap of joy. The additional two mentioned in Ayurvedic texts are the sheen of the skin and the shadow on the ground.

By examining these traps and then observing society, one can see how different people are caught in different traps according to their habitual patterns. These different traps are nothing but the different fields of consciousness through which the mind operates. The slightest trace of obsession with any of these fields will render the individual a slave to that field. On the other hand, if one is alert to this tendency, one can maintain a detachment from these fields of projecting consciousness. Then, by developing the appropriate skills, one can use the energy inherent in these fields to fulfill one's deeper needs.

Hatha yoga provides the appropriate means for yoking the energy of these fields. The practice of asana with the controlled intake of pure foods gives control of the *annamaya kosha. Kriya, pranayama, bandha,* and *mudra* harness the energies of the remaining fields. When all these energies are harnessed and brought under voluntary control, the internal process of *laya* (absorption) may begin. The link to the internal process is *pratyahara*. This evolves later into *dharana, dhyana,* and *samadhi* (or *nadanusandana,* as it is termed in the hatha yogic texts). The remaining two layers, the sheen of the skin and the shadow on the ground, are utilized for diagnostic purposes. A good sheen on the skin demonstrates that the inner fire *(agni)* is functioning properly. *Agni* is responsible for the healthy functioning of all the inner fields.

Skillful reading of the shadow can reveal things about the individual's future. Reflection on the nature of these inner fields will make it clear that activity imposed by the mind on the body will not bring these energies under voluntary control. This control can only be achieved through natural patterns of behavior. This means one must start with preliminary movements like squatting, lunging, and various movements of the arms and hands, in order to uncover the natural patterns of motion latent in the physical form.

5
One Hundred and Eight Marmas: The Vital Junctions (Points)

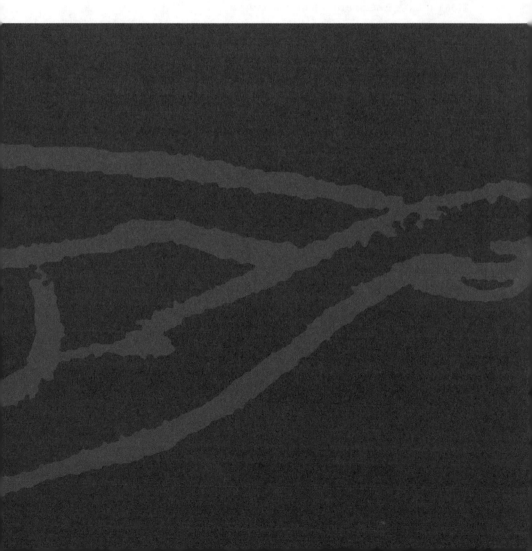

There are 108 vital junctions spread over the surface of the body and its limbs. They appear at the intersections of different muscular patterns, joints, arteries, veins, nerves, and subtle energy currents. These are the vulnerable areas or key points to different energetic centers of organic activity.

The word *marma* is derived from the root *mrt-*, which means "death." *Marmas* were first observed to be vulnerable areas and have been utilized in *Kalaripayyat,* the Indian martial art (in the science of striking and reviving), and in Ayurvedic therapy (in massage). They also respond to different patterns of muscular use, movement, and breathing. Each *marma* relates to specific *vayus* (the different *pranas*), *doshas* (humors), *dhatus* (tissues), and *shrotas* (channels).

This system was devised and developed by the great South Indian sage Agastya and is highly recommended by two ancient texts: the *Yogayajnavalkya Samhita* and the *Vasishta Samhita* (or the *Yoga Kanda* of Vasishta). At the beginning of the chapter on meditation *(dhyana),* Yajnavalkya states:

Only after understanding the marmas-thana, the junction of nadi and the location of vayu, must one proceed with the understanding of atma.

Yogayajnavalkya Samhita IX.4

The *marmas* of this system should not be confused with the points of Chinese acupuncture, although many parallels may be found in the two systems. Twelve of the 108 *marma* junctions are said to be of vital importance, while the other ninety-six are termed medial life centers. The twelve central life centers are situated between the center of the perineal floor *(yonisthana)* and the crown of the head *(adhipati),* and they include the seven chakras.

The ninety-six medial life centers are peripheral. Thirty-two govern the nerves and soft tissues, while sixty-four directly affect the blood and blood vessels. The ninety-six peripheral centers are in charge of the eight *nadis* (channels) that carry the life force through the peripheral areas and feed into the central channels. These are: two channels from the eyes to their corresponding big toes, two from the ears to their corresponding big toes, the channel from the throat to the head of the genitals, the channel from the neck to the anus, and the two belt channels that encircle the abdomen, one from left to right, the other from right to left. When good peripheral activity is achieved, these channels are cleared and the energy flows through them without obstruction. This energy then feeds into the central channels.

Correct activation of these *marmas* enhances all these functions, while incorrect activation will damage them. For example, the junctions in the wrists, ankles, and neck govern the tendons and connective tissue throughout the body and are therefore responsible for flexibility. Failure to correctly activate these junctions often results in injury to other joints and tissues. The *marmasthana* information makes it clear that the appropriate use of the arms and legs increases circulation and space and support for the joints, while incorrect use decreases these, which can eventually result in injury, both to the joints and to the organs that correspond to those joints.

It is through the system of *marmas* that the natural patterns of bodily activity can be discovered and the energy mastered without injury. When the map of *marmas* is memorized and put to work in the practice of asanas, *kriya, bandha, pranayama,* and *mudra* benefits will quickly accrue. The *marmas* not only affect the physiological functions but also exercise great influence over the pranic force in the thirteen *nadis*. This force then pierces the seven chakras (subtle inner energy centers), rendering them passive. With the chakras passive, the *prana* is no longer dissipated, and the intense energy that results is termed the *shakti*. At the same time that the yoga practices move closer to meditation, the *marmas* all over the body are brought under voluntary control. When this level of control is reached, the *marmas* can be closed at will, turning the whole surface of the body into protective armor. This further conserves the dissipation of energy and increases the *shakti* (inner latent power).

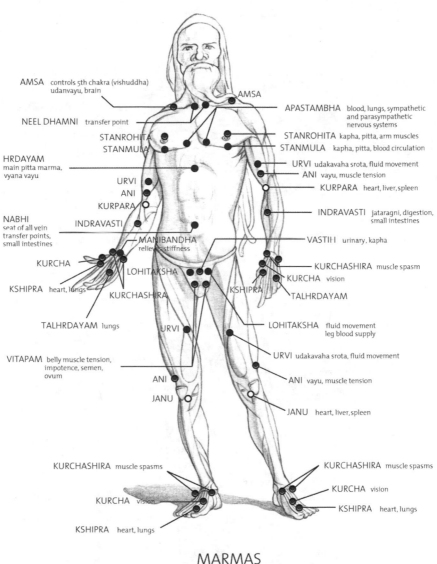

AMSA controls 5th chakra (vishuddha)
udanvayu, brain

AMSA

APASTAMBHA blood, lungs, sympathetic
and parasympathetic
nervous systems

NEEL DHAMNI transfer point

STANROHITA kapha, pitta, arm muscles

STANROHITA
STANMULA

STANMULA kapha, pitta, blood circulation

HRDAYAM
main pitta marma,
vyana vayu

URVI udakavaha srota, fluid movement

ANI vayu, muscle tension

URVI

KURPARA heart, liver, spleen

ANI

KURPARA

INDRAVASTI jataragni, digestion,
small intestines

NABHI
seat of all vein
transfer points,
small intestines

INDRAVASTI

MANIBANDHA
relieves stiffness

VASTIH urinary, kapha

KURCHA

LOHITAKSHA

KURCHASHIRA muscle spasm

KSHIPRA heart, lungs

KURCHA vision

KURCHASHIRA

KSHIPRA

TALHRDAYAM

TALHRDAYAM lungs

LOHITAKSHA fluid movement
leg blood supply

VITAPAM belly muscle tension,
impotence, semen,
ovum

URVI udakavaha srota, fluid movement

ANI

ANI vayu, muscle tension

JANU

JANU heart, liver, spleen

KURCHASHIRA muscle spasms

KURCHASHIRA muscle spasms

KURCHA vision

KURCHA vision

KSHIPRA heart, lungs

KSHIPRA heart, lungs

MARMAS

 soft tissue, large muscles, connective tissue, ligaments, tendons and sinews

glandular and circulatory systems: blood, lymph and secretions

bones, joints, sutures and nerves

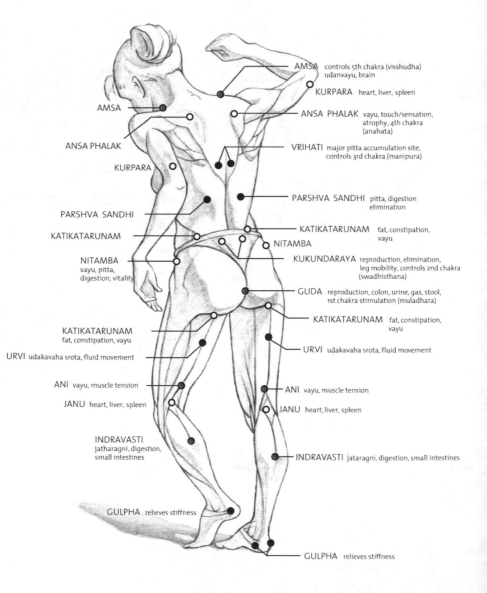

AMSA controls 5th chakra (visshudha) udanvayu, brain

KURPARA heart, liver, spleen

AMSA

ANSA PHALAK vayu, touch/sensation, atrophy, 4th chakra (anahata)

ANSA PHALAK

VRIHATI major pitta accumulation site, controls 3rd chakra (manipura)

KURPARA

PARSHVA SANDHI pitta, digestion elimination

KATIKATARUNAM fat, constipation, vayu

PARSHVA SANDHI

NITAMBA

KATIKATARUNAM

KUKUNDARAYA reproduction, elimination, leg mobility, controls 2nd chakra (swadhisthana)

NITAMBA vayu, pitta, digestion, vitality

GUDA reproduction, colon, urine, gas, stool, 1st chakra stimulation (muladhara)

KATIKATARUNAM fat, constipation, vayu

KATIKATARUNAM fat, constipation, vayu

URVI udakavaha srota, fluid movement

URVI udakavaha srota, fluid movement

ANI vayu, muscle tension

ANI vayu, muscle tension

JANU heart, liver, spleen

JANU heart, liver, spleen

INDRAVASTI jatharagni, digestion, small intestines

INDRAVASTI jataragni, digestion, small intestines

GULPHA relieves stiffness

GULPHA relieves stiffness

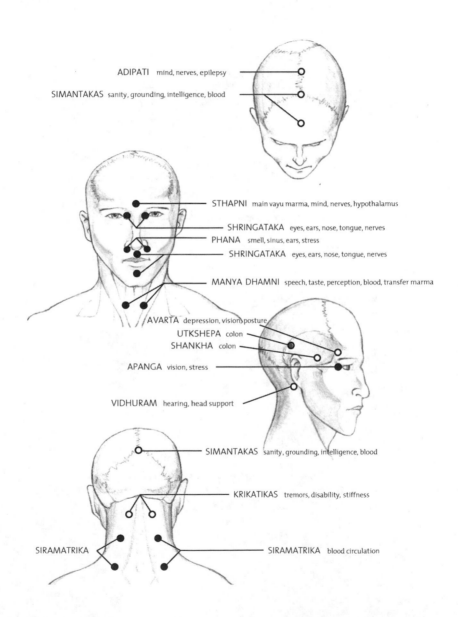

ADIPATI mind, nerves, epilepsy

SIMANTAKAS sanity, grounding, intelligence, blood

STHAPNI main vayu marma, mind, nerves, hypothalamus

SHRINGATAKA eyes, ears, nose, tongue, nerves

PHANA smell, sinus, ears, stress

SHRINGATAKA eyes, ears, nose, tongue, nerves

MANYA DHAMNI speech, taste, perception, blood, transfer marma

AVARTA depression, vision, posture

UTKSHEPA colon

SHANKHA colon

APANGA vision, stress

VIDHURAM hearing, head support

SIMANTAKAS sanity, grounding, intelligence, blood

KRIKATIKAS tremors, disability, stiffness

SIRAMATRIKA

SIRAMATRIKA blood circulation

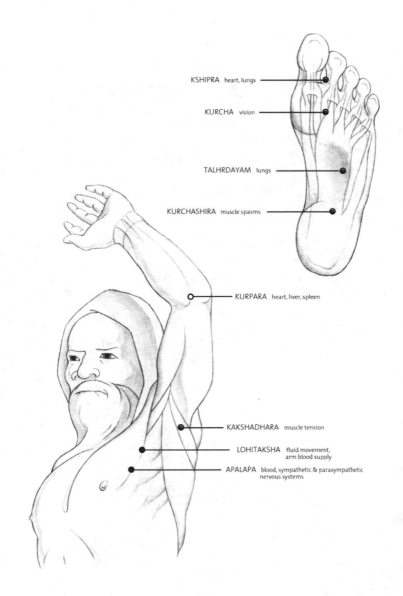

KSHIPRA heart, lungs

KURCHA vision

TALHRDAYAM lungs

KURCHASHIRA muscle spasms

KURPARA heart, liver, spleen

KAKSHADHARA muscle tension

LOHITAKSHA fluid movement, arm blood supply

APALAPA blood, sympathetic & parasympathetic nervous systems

6
The Chakras

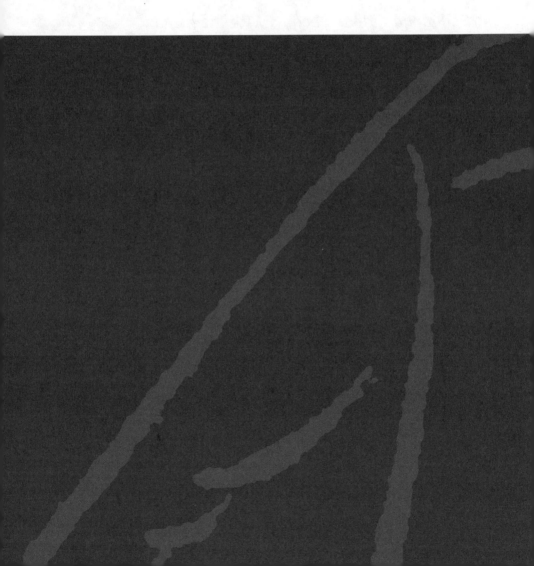

Before entering a discussion on the chakra system one should consider the three different levels of yogic practices *(yoganga sadhana)*. These are *bahiranga* (external), *antaranga* (internal), and *paramantaranga* (supreme). This third stage reveals the existence of god and the soul in humans and leads to the connection of the *jivatma* (individual self) and *paramatma* (god).

Bahiranga sadhana begins with the *yamas* and ends with *pratyahara.* Hatha yoga only stresses one *yama—mitahara* (controlled intake of pure food)—and one *niyama— ahimsa* (nonviolence)—that must be brought to life through the practice of asana, *kriya, bandha, pranayama, mudra,* and *pratyahara. Bahiranga sadhana* cures all the diseases of the body that are apparent to the senses. *Dharana, dhyana,* and *samadhi,* the other three limbs, belong to *antaranga sadhana* and together are referred to as *samyama.*

Antaranga sadhana works on the mind, the brain, and the heart *(hrdayam).* The *hrdayam* should not be confused with the physical organ that pumps blood, but is located in the *anahata chakra.* The workings of the *hrdayam* are not directly perceptible to the senses but are responsible for the cure of all diseases related to the mind, the brain, and the heart.

Paramantaranga sadhana is *dharma megha samadhi,* the final stepping-stone to *kaivalya* (isolation) as described by the sage Patanjali that corresponds exactly to the term *kevala kumbhaka* (used in the texts of hatha yoga). *Kevala kumbhaka* (spontaneous cessation of breath) is the final outcome of asana, *kriya, bandha, pranayama*—the *sahita kumbhaka* (imposed cessation of breath), *mudra,* and *nadanusandana.*

The *hrdayam* is supported by the seven chakras. These supports for the *hrdayam* are also termed *nadi granthis* (knots within the central channel of *sushumna*) since they act as blockages to the *shakti* in the ordinary individual. The mind or *manas* has its seat in the hole of the heart in the *anahata chakra* and is only inferior to the *jivatma* (*antaryami,* the indweller) and the *paramatma.* The *manas* can understand joy and sorrow, which is not possible to the senses and organs of action.

The seven chakras supporting the *hrdayam* are:

Muladhara between the anus and the root of the genitals
Swadhisthana at the origin of the genitals
Manipura at the navel

Anahata at the heart
Vishuddha at the base of the throat
Ajna between the eyebrows
Sahasrara at the crown of the head.

These seven chakras are active in three ways: *avritti* (dissipating motion) due to *puraka, rechaka,* and *kumbhaka* (inhalation, exhalation, and their retention); *parivritti* (spiraling) as a result of the proper control of the three *bandhas;* and *samavritti* (even rhythm) due to the variation in the length of *rechaka kumbhaka* (exhalation and exhalation retention) during *pranayama* (this refers to the thirty-second verse of Patanjali's *Samadhi Pada*).

These seven chakras in themselves are not perceptible to the senses or emotions, but their activities can be perceived by the mind, just like the experience of joy and sorrow. The activity of the seven chakras is brought to a complete halt during *kevala kumbhaka,* which is the voluntary stopping of respiration.

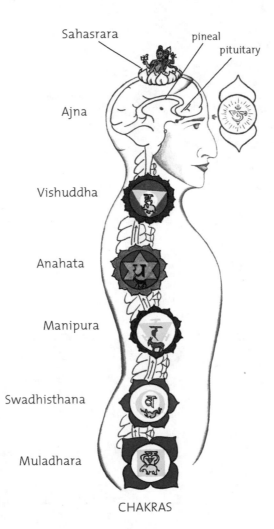

Sahasrara

pineal
pituitary

Ajna

Vishuddha

Anahata

Manipura

Swadhisthana

Muladhara

CHAKRAS

7
The Ten Vayus (Winds or Motivators of the Pranic Force)

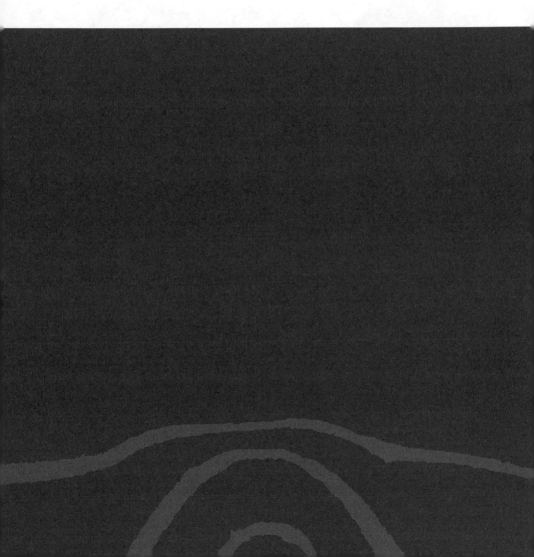

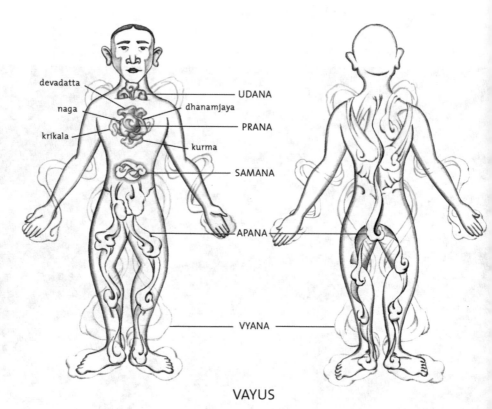

devadatta

naga

krikala

UDANA

dhanamjaya

PRANA

kurma

SAMANA

APANA

VYANA

VAYUS

Free movement of the ten *vayus* (winds) leads to a strong mind and body, as well as to longevity. The main *vayus* are *prana, apana, samana, udana,* and *vyana,* and they carry out the main functions in the different areas of the body. The remaining five are termed the *nagadi vayus* (sub-winds), and are responsible for the relief of the different sorts of tension that arise in the body due to the stresses of life. The locations and functions of the primary vayus are as follows:

Pranavayu

The main seat is in the heart *(hrdayam),* but it is also located at the tip of the nose, in the navel, and in the big toes. Its color is green, and its nature is hot. It is responsible for inhalation and for the separation of solid, liquid, and gaseous food substances within the duodenum. It also maintains the health of the organs in the head region.

Apanavayu (the downward moving wind)

The main seat is the anus, but it is also located at the base of the neck and the spine, along with the whole of the back and the heels. It is responsible for all types of elimination, including exhalation, defecation, urination, ejaculation, the holding of the child within the womb during pregnancy, and also delivery. During the passage out of the womb, a type of *apanavayu* causes the child to forget its previous births. Its color is black. When this wind is weakened because of incorrect lifestyle it can cause major health problems.

Samanavayu (the equalizer)

The main seat is the navel, but it is also located at the whorl of the hair. Its color is white. This current is responsible for the assimilation of the essences of food as well as the electromagnetic currents from the process of respiration and the assimilation of thought patterns.

Udanavayu (the upward moving wind)

The main seat is at the base of the throat, but it is also located in the heart, the uvula, the third eye, and the crown of the head. Its color is red. It is responsible for carrying the power upward within the central channels (of the *sushumna* and *vajrini nadis*). This wind contributes most to the practice of the three *bandhas—uddiyana, mula,* and *jalandhara*—including the practice of *nauli kriya* (the rotation of the rectus abdominis muscle). When this wind is abused through incorrect practice it leads to deep-seated psychological and physiological illnesses that damage the endocrine system. The control of this current should be achieved without imposition by using the intuitive intelligence.

Vyanavayu (the circulating wind)

The seat is the skin all over the body. Its color is that of the rainbow. It is responsible for circulation and for the delivery of all types of food essence to the different parts of the body.

The *nagadi vayus* (sub-*vayus* that are situated within and around the heart) are:

Kurma (the tortoise)

Its seat is directly under the heart and it is responsible for blinking.

Krikara (the partridge)

Its seat is on either side of the heart and it is responsible for sneezing, hunger, and belching.

Devadatta (the gift of the gods)

Its seat is slightly above the heart and it is responsible for yawning.

Naga (the serpent)

Its seat is in the center of the heart and it is responsible for the intuitive free movements of the body's limbs, acting as a release mechanism for *prana shakti,* which lives in the skin.

Dhanamjaya (the giver of victory)

This wind is all-pervasive and is responsible for the movement of sound throughout the whole body. It is present in the body during life and after death, when it causes the decomposition of the body. Its seat is in the center of the heart.

These ten winds are merely the different functions of the one pranic force responding to the different demands of life. Through the proper practices of yoga all these winds and functions are strengthened, rendering the body healthy and strong. This frees the pranic force from excessive demands related to the maintenance of the gross structure.

8
The Thirteen Nadis
(Subtle Energy Flows)

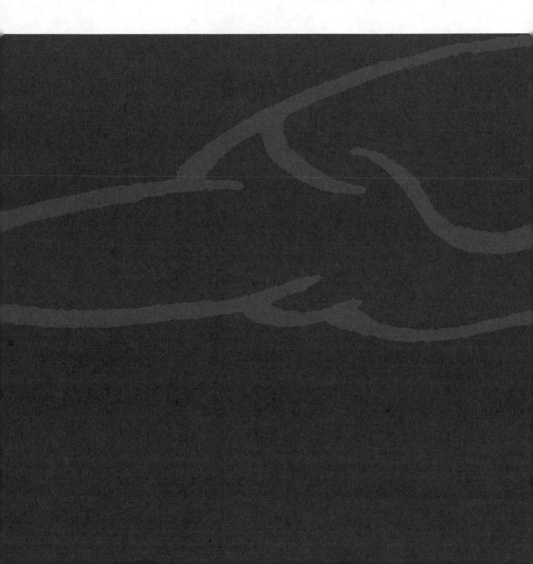

According to yogic anatomy, the *vayus* are carried through a network of *nadis*. These number 72,000 and spread throughout the whole body. Of these 72,000, yoga is only concerned with thirteen. These thirteen are *ida, pingala, sushumna, alambusha* (or *saraswati*), *vajrini, gandhari, hastijiva, pusha, yashashvini, kuhu, shankini, varuni,* and *vishvodhara*. These *nadis* are the most important trans-porters of the pranic force or *vayu*.

These *nadis* all stem from the bulb *(kanda)*, which hangs from the *sushumna* like a jewel on a thread slightly below the *manipura chakra*.

The *ida nadi,* channel of the moon, is connected to the left nostril and is responsible for the cooling of the entire system and the supply of energy to the heart. The direction of this energy is to the south and west. The *pingala nadi* is the channel of the sun, gives rise to heat in the body, and is connected to the right nostril. It supplies the brain, and its direction is to the north and east. The *sushumna nadi* con-sists of three flows—the upward *(arohan),* the downward *(avarohan),* and the thrusting *(vajrini)*. These correspond to the governing, functioning, and thrusting meridians of the Chinese system. The downward flow is also termed *alam-busha* (or *saraswati) nadi,* the channel of the tongue. The tongue also acts as a bridge between the central and peripheral *nadis*. The *sushumna nadi* is often referred to as *smashana* (the burning grounds), which reveals its true identity as the bearer of fire.

The remaining eight *nadis* carry the pranic force to the peripheral areas of the body. *Gandhari* travels from the *kanda* to the left eye and also to the big toe of the left foot. *Hastijiva* travels from the *kanda* to the right eye and also to the big toe of the right foot. *Pusha* travels from the *kanda* to the right ear and also to the big toe of the right foot. *Yashashvini* travels from the *kanda* to the left ear and also to the big toe of the left foot. *Kuhu* travels from the *kanda* to the throat and also to the head of the genitals. *Shankini* connects the neck and the anus through the *kanda*. *Varuni* and *vishvodhara* are the two belt channels, the former running from left to right, the latter from right to left. Both start from the *kanda* and terminate in the *kanda* on the opposite side.

If the movement of *vayu* is disturbed in these *nadis* by the overgrowth of muscles or other causes, the outcome is imbalance. There is a warning in some texts (including those of the late Sri T. Krishnamacharya, the father of present-day yoga) that people must refrain from repetitive and one-sided activity. Where one type of movement is continuously repeated throughout a practice session, it leads to an overgrowth of those muscle groups that are being repeatedly used. This leads to the obstruction of the movement of the pranic force, which gives rise to a host of diseases while causing the mind to become fixed and mechanical. However, when the practice of asanas is mastered, it renders fluid both the mind and the pranic force.

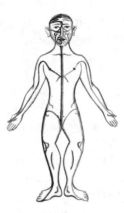

ida & pingala

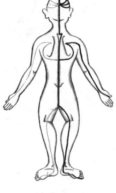

ida & pingala

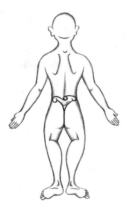

vishvodhara

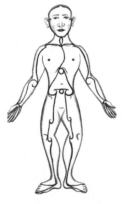

gandhari & hastijiva

NADIS

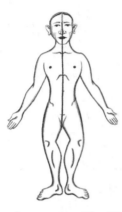

sushumna, saraswati & vajrini

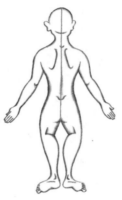

sushumna

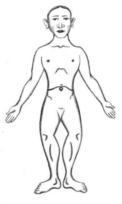

varuni

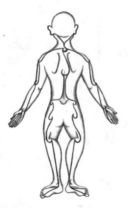

pusha & yashashvini

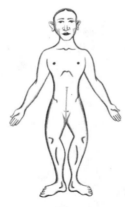

kuhu

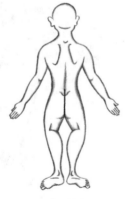

shankini

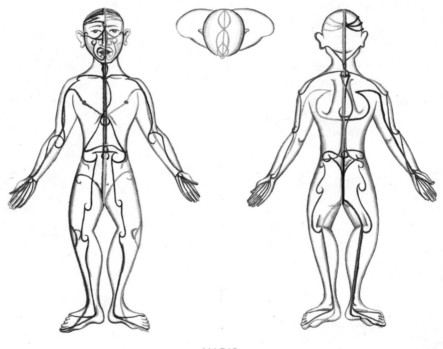

NADIS

9
The Tongue

Of all the *jnanendriyas* and the *karmendriyas,* the tongue
plays the most complex and significant role. It is the organ
of perception for taste, and the organ of action for speech.
All the major organs, nerves, ligaments, tendons, sinews,
and sutures are under the influence of the tongue. The
hatha yoga texts state that there is no asana like *siddhasana,* no *kumbhaka* like *kevala,* no *mudra* like *khechari,*
and no *laya* like *nadanusandana.* What concerns us here is
the importance given to the *khechari mudra* (the moving-
in-space gesture). This deals with the placement of the
tongue appropriate to the different practices of hatha yoga.

The tongue is the switch between the gross and the subtle,
and between the central and peripheral energy systems. It
plays a great role in the voluntary control of the sixteen
sinews and the seven sutures throughout the yogic practices. There are sixteen sinews *(kandara)*—two in each arm,
two in each leg, four in the throat, and four in the neck.
Those in the arms and legs extend to the tips of the fingers
and toes. Those in the throat pass through the heart and
terminate in the generative organ, and those in the back
terminate in the anus. Of the seven fibrous sutures *(shivani),* five are found in the cranium, one in the tongue, and
one in the penis or the clitoris.

Through the connection between the tongue and the
sinews, one can influence and direct the movement of the
body parts using pranic force rather than heavy muscular
activity. Through the tongue's influence over the sutures,
one can increase or decrease the inner space of the skull in
order to adjust the brain and its function during refined
practice of *pranasamyama.*

A set of daily exercises has been prescribed for the cultivation of the tongue's energy. These are extremely important

even if one is not interested in undergoing the prolonged process involved in achieving *khechari mudra* (which requires the guidance of a guru). These preliminary exercises consist of the massaging and stretching or "milking" of the tongue. Inserting the three middle fingers into the mouth, massage the root of the tongue. Next, use the thumbs to massage the sides and bottom of the tongue, including the fraenum (the sinew attached to the tongue). Then take the thumbs and massage the roof of the mouth, including the hard and soft palates and the uvula.

At first this practice will feel a little strange, but this reaction will soon disappear. There will be some thick salivation, which will grow thinner as the energy begins to clarify. After the massage, take a thin, clean towel, take hold of the tip of the tongue with the thumb and index fingers of both hands, and then pull the tongue down below the tip of the chin, up toward the bridge of the nose, and then from side to side. This milking should be done thirty to fifty times in the morning before practice. Finally, hold the towel with the three middle fingers and wipe the surface of the tongue clean until the tongue regains its natural deep pink color. By milking the tongue in this way it is surprisingly easy to release the stiffness of the inner organs as well as those of the limbs.

There is a milder form of *khechari mudra,* termed *jiva bandha* (lock of the soul). Every practitioner can and should use this during the practice of yoga.

There are four distinct points located on the hard and soft palates where different energies can be brought under control and directed by the placement of the tip of the tongue. These points correspond to the different elements operating in the body.

1. For the practice of asana, the tip of the tongue should always be placed against the palate behind the root of the front upper teeth, though without actually touching the teeth. This is the seat of the element wind. Holding the tongue at this point makes the movement of the breath much deeper and the motion of the body smoother and lighter.

2. Placing the tip of the tongue against the center of the roof of the palate increases the heating process in the body, since this is the seat of fire in the mouth.

3. Sometimes the surface of the tongue and mouth becomes dry due to excess heat. At such times, one should roll the tongue back further and place the tip of the tongue at the edge of the soft palate. This increases moisture throughout the body because this is the seat of water in the mouth, and this is accompanied by an increase in energy.

4. When there is an experience of instability in the mind or the body, one should push the tip of the tongue toward the tip of the uvula while at the same time contracting the uvula toward the tongue. When the two tips meet the mind and the limbs will gain stability since the tip of the uvula is the seat of earth within the back of the mouth. When the two tips touch, one will experience a firm contraction directly above the center of the perineal floor, the seat of the element earth in the body.

5. The fifth point is the seat of ether, which is situated between the eyebrows, the location of the third eye. This is the point used in *khechari mudra,* which will not be dealt with in this book.

When the practice of *jiva bandha* is refined, the tongue will move of its own accord to these energy points to provide the necessary quality according to the needs of the practice at that moment. All these variations provide a necessary seal to prevent the leakage of energy.

This concludes the theoretical information necessary for a well-grounded and rewarding practice of hatha yoga. Deprived of this, the mind remains dull and blind to the energies awakened by the practices of yoga. This information should be received in such a way that it can be used spontaneously by the mind in action.

10
Asanas: The Tools

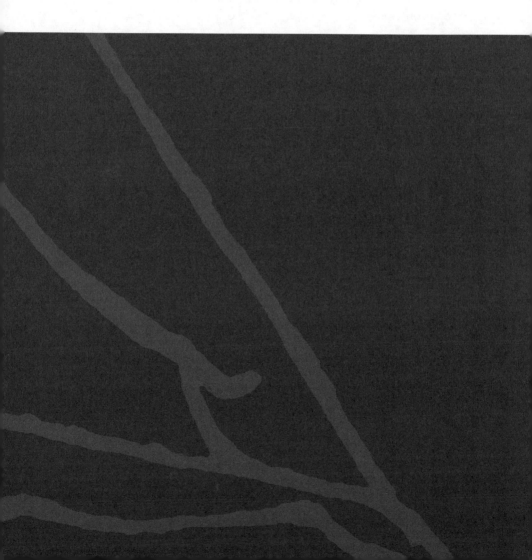

When put to use, the theoretical information presented will cultivate the *yamas* (restraints) and *niyamas* (observances), which are the basis of all yogic activities. The *yamas* and *niyamas* prepare the mind for the practice of asana. However, asana, third in the order of the *ashtanga* (eight limbs), plays a great role in enlivening the first two. This occurs because in the work of asana one is able to observe in action one's own patterns of behavior, both conscious and unconscious.

If the mind is dull or sleeping, the activity of asana forces it to awaken. A well-tuned mind is free from any type of thinking, and yet is fully aware of everything that happens. It is this combination of qualities that enables the mind to be spontaneous and fluid. To cultivate this, in the Shadow School, the asanas are practiced with a number of different rhythms and energetic patterns. These progress from fluid, through static-dynamic, to stillness with interchanging patterns of spiral, circular, and linear movement. These are arranged in three phases—the prelude, *asana-vinyasa,* and conclusion. Together they involve the full curriculum of *bahiranga sadhana* (asana, *kriya, bandha, pranayama, mudra, pratyahara*).

There are three fixed sequences in the Shadow School, the primary, intermediate, and advanced sequence, so named according to the level and type of activity involved.

1. *Balakrama*—Stepping into Strength
2. *Chaya Yoddha Sancalanam*—Churning of the Shadow Warrior
3. *Karttikeya Mandala*—Garland of Light

These three levels of practice accommodate the various levels of student *(sadhaka),* which are three: mild, medium, or intense. According to his or her individual capacity, the student is taken through the preludes to the different levels of asana to the threshold of *antaranga* (internal) and *para-mantaranga* (supreme) *sadhanas.*

How can these sequences of asanas possibly bring the practitioner to such a point?

The first thing one should examine is how the innumerable variations of the five body positions of forward, sideward, and backward bends, twists, and balances bring about different states of transformation. This is achieved through their influence over the five major winds that are responsible for the basic life functions.

A forward bend like *paśchimottanasana* reduces the capacity for inhalation while increasing exhalation, causing the body to become light. It restricts the movement of *prana vayu* while facilitating the movement of *apana vayu*. This is brought about by the contraction of the lower abdomen and the increased pressure on the area of the rectum and toward the heels. At the same time, the head presses the energy from the base of the neck to the anus, the main seat of *apana vayu*, forcing the *prana* to enter the *sushumna* (central channel).

A side bend like *ardha chandrasana* restricts both inhalation and exhalation, while a back bend like *urdhva dha-nurasana* restricts exhalation and increases inhalation. In the latter case, the resulting expansion of the body creates more inner space and intensifies *agni*. Twists and balances also restrict *prana* and lengthen *apana*. In addition, they force into action the other three *vayus (samana, udana,* and *vyana),* because of the acute pressure on the area of the navel. When one considers the above information, it is clear why such importance is placed on making exhalation twice as long as inhalation. With correct exhalation, the mind is brought to a state of surrender, empty of thought. It is of great importance that we understand the relationship between inner and outer work in practice. The gross body continuously influences the subtle currents. With this knowledge we can use the physical form, our chief instrument, with intelligence and care but without pampering it.

The type of breathing that should be adopted during the practice of asana is also important. This is a simple form of *ujjayi*. The breath is slightly restrained through the narrowing of the base of the throat and the application of the three *bandhas*. This causes a gentle hissing sound behind the heart. This accompanies the increase in *sadhaka pitta*, which is located there and is responsible for the control of cardiac temperature. The power within the breath should arise from the proper placement of the body and fluid movement. This is only possible when each position is executed on its point of balance without overuse or underuse of the limbs. If the body's point of balance is maintained throughout the practice, whether holding a position or moving between positions, many things are gained. The tissues of the body gain even toning, the breath becomes smooth and fluid, and the mind will be void of all thoughts. This is the unimposed state of *dharana* (concentration), the first step toward meditation.

If practitioners work in this direction they will arrive at a point where they understand both the inside and the outside of the asanas. For teachers, it is important that they are capable of demonstrating what they teach, but also that they understand which asanas are good for what type of ailments and how they should be applied with regard to duration and breathing.

Good demonstrations are required, but without the knowledge of the curative aspects of *asanas, kriyas, bandhas, pranayamas,* and *mudras,* people will not benefit from these practices and the science of yoga will be lost to future generations.

At the same time, theoretical information not worked with in practice may bring certification, but will not yield results in the real world.

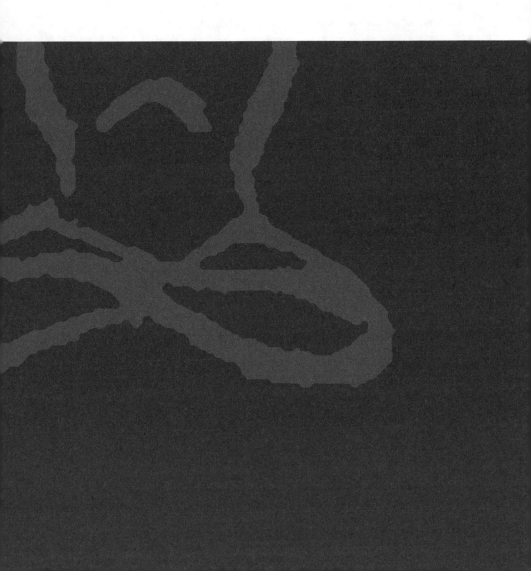

11
Nauli Kriya

Nauli, lauliki, nauliki, and *chalani* are all synonyms for *nauli kriya. Nauli kriya* (the churning process) is the king of the *shatkarmas,* the six acts that are frequently described as cleansing processes, but fulfill a more important function in *yoga sadhana.*

The *pancha karmas* (the five acts of Ayurveda) are more appropriate for cleansing, and should be done before the *yoga sadhana* is begun. The *shatkarmas* are used mainly for gaining control over involuntary actions. Here we will only deal with *nauli kriya,* since its use is an integral part of *bahiranga sadhana.* The other five acts should only be used according to individual needs over a short period of time. Information about them can be found in most hatha yoga texts.

Nauli kriya involves a churning of the abdominal viscera by the rectus abdominis muscle, to draw the inner heat from the abdominal fluids. This image of churning was borrowed from the circular motions of the fire stick of the Vedic fire rituals. The mastery of this process requires the acquisition of the three *bandhas.* When *uddiyana* is complete the other two *bandhas* follow spontaneously and *nauli* becomes accessible.

The practice of *nauli* cannot be learned from books. One needs to work with a teacher who has mastered it and clearly understands its function.

Its main use is at the bridging point between asana and *pranayama* and in the practice of *shakti chalana mudra* (the churning or raising of power). The practice of *nauli kriya* is always combined with *kapalabhati* or *bhastrika pranayama,* and is performed during *bahir kumbhaka* (external retention of the breath).

If practiced daily, the standard number of rotations is five hundred to a thousand at one sitting. More can be done but this is sufficient for the average practitioner. To reach this number of rotations requires about fifteen minutes. The rotations should be done from left to right first, and then from right to left within each set. The number of rotations should be increased slowly without sacrificing thoroughness. The combined practice of *bhastrika pranayama, uddiyana bandha,* and *nauli kriya* helps the practitioner gain control over the three *doshas—vata, pitta,* and *kapha.*

Nauli kriya increases the movement of wind, feeding the inner fire while stabilizing its flame. For this reason, it is called the king of the six acts. With the consistent practice of *nauli kriya,* the body becomes light and firm, free from energetic obstructions.

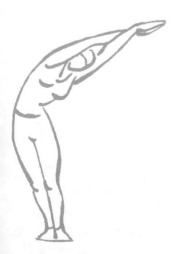

12
Pranayama

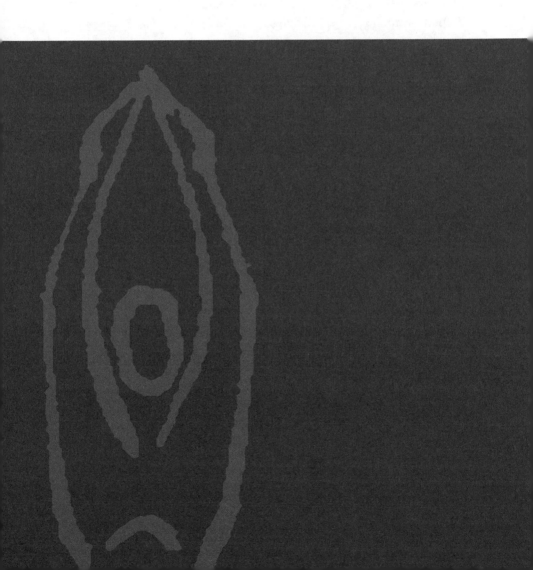

The word *pranayama* has layers of meaning. According to the science of yoga, *prana*, usually translated as "life force," is a subtle form of energy that exists in all living beings until their death. This energy controls all the life functions within the body.

Prana should not be mistaken for the air involved in the physical process of breathing. Nor should it be confused with the *jivatman* (the indwelling soul). *Ayama,* the second half of the compound, refers to a lengthening or prolonging process. The "lengthening" of the *prana* implies the idea of conservation, that the energy is in some ways limited and must be made to last longer by a process of restraint. This is achieved by regulating the pattern of respiration, which maximizes the potential of this energy. This is accomplished by manipulating the four phases of the respiration process:

1. *Puraka*—inhalation
2. *Antara kumbhaka*—retention of inhalation
3. *Rechaka*—exhalation
4. *Bhaya kumbhaka*—retention of exhalation

These four phases can be practiced with even or uneven ratios. The even ratios are called *samavritti,* while the uneven ones are referred to as *vishamavritti pranayama.* If the counting of the length of the three phases is done through the use of mantras it is termed *samantrakam.* When counting is done with numbers only, it is called *amantrakam* or *tantrikam.*

There is one type of *pranayama* that goes beyond these four phases. This is termed *kevala kumbhaka,* the voluntary and complete cessation of respiration. In this state, the pranic force is completely isolated within a closed circuit. This is the highest form of *pranayama* and is the natural outcome of well-conducted respiratory regulation. Most hatha yoga texts list ten different types of *pranayama* for the regulation of the breath:

1. *Suryabhedana*—piercing the sun
2. *Ujjayi*—the victorious breath
3. *Nadi shodhana*—cleansing of the channels
4. *Sitkari*—cooling breath
5. *Shitali*—cooling breath
6. *Bramhari*—humming
7. *Lahari* or *Plavini*—floating
8. *Kapalabhati*—shining of the skull
9. *Bhastri*—bellows
10. *Murcha*—swooning

The *Hatha Pradipika* of Svatmarama Yogendra lists only
eight *(lahari* and *murcha* are excluded). Sri T.
Krishnamacharya, in addition to these two, also excludes
bramhari. He considered the effects of those three *pranaya-mas* to be purely physical, short lasting and tending to
cause spiritual retardation.

Of the seven remaining *pranayamas, suryabhedana, ujjayi,*
and *nadi shodhana* are to spiritually uplift the individual.
They must be practiced well for a long time before their
fruits are experienced, but their beneficial effects are long
lasting. *Sitkari, shitali, kapalabhati,* and *bhastri* are purely
physical but also beneficial.

The practice of *pranayama* is conducted utilizing the three
modes of *anuloma, viloma,* and *pratiloma.* These modes are
given to the student according to individual requirements.
They help to regulate the mind and maintain the right
direction in this demanding discipline. Before engaging in
the practice of *pranayama* one should gain control of the
basic asanas. Without this, *pranayama* is not possible. Of all
the asanas, *padmasana* (when performed with all three
bandhas) is the most suitable for *pranayama.*

The movement of *vayu* through the nostrils is regulated
using the right hand. The index and middle fingers are bent
into the base of the right thumb. The tip of the thumb is

then made to touch the tips of the ring and little fingers; this gesture is termed *mrigi mudra* (gesture of the deer) or *omkara* (the gesture of om). The hand is then applied to the nostrils so that the thumb regulates the right influx while the tip of the ring and little fingers control the left influx. The tips of the thumb and fingers are placed near the middle of the nose at the edge of the septum and gently pull the skin toward the tip of the nose. The *marma* called *phana* (the hood) is located where the fingers touch and governs the area of the brain responsible for respiration.

Of the eight *pranayamas* recommended above, *suryabhedana* should be practiced first. Only when *suryabhedana* has been mastered will the other *pranayamas* yield significant benefits. This *pranayama* is responsible for removing all the impurities in the body that obstruct or hamper the circulation of heat and light. The correct application of the three *bandhas* constitutes the foundation of *pranayama* practice. *Mulabandha* is maintained during the entire practice; *jalandhara* is introduced at the end of inhalation and is maintained during its retention, the exhalation, and the retention of the exhalation. *Uddiyana* is introduced at the beginning of exhalation and is maintained through its entire length as well as during the retention that follows. The modifications in the three *bandhas* regulate the rhythmic patterns of *pranayama* by increasing or decreasing the pressures within the different body cavities. It should be noted that the use of *uddiyana bandha* during the initial stages of *pranayama* practice may cause discomfort in the navel area, the liver, the spleen, and the solar plexus. These discomforts slowly ease and finally disappear with consistent practice.

Ujjayi, with *anuloma* or *viloma* modes, is used to cleanse the breathing passages. *Ujjayi* in *pratiloma* mode is a combination of these two. The regular practice of this *pranayama* helps in maintaining the health of the nose, lungs, and breathing passages and helps in drawing the mind towards a steady state. *Anuloma* is effective in the treatment of diseases of the nasal passages, while *viloma* cures diseases of the throat and tonsils.

Nadi shodhana pranayama cleanses the arterial vessels that flow from the heart. *Kapalabhati* dries up the excess phlegm within the skull, while *bhastrika pranayama* gets rid of the excess phlegm from the lungs and the rest of the body. *Sitkari* and *shitali pranayamas* remove excess heat from the body, while *sitkari* is also responsible for the removal of poisons from the blood.

With the exception of *suryabhedana, ujjayi* (in *anuloma, viloma,* and *pratiloma* modes), and *nadi shodhana pranayamas,* all the other *pranayamas* are only used for therapeutic purposes. These three *pranayamas* also have therapeutic effects, but their main role is to regulate the fluctuations of the mind and annihilate habits of attachment.

13
Mudras

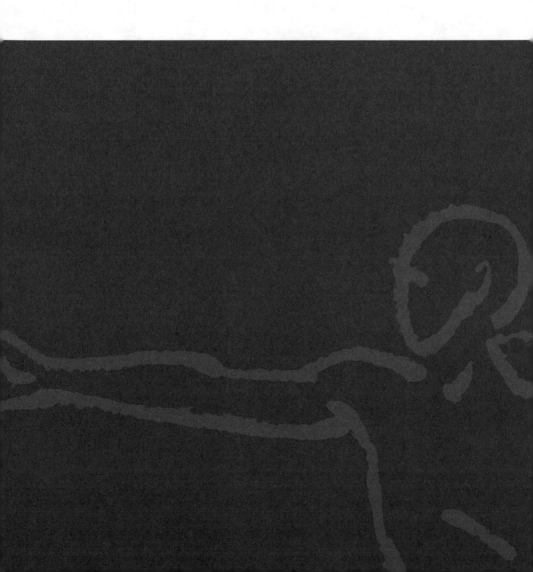

The word *mudra* describes a seal or hermetic isolation. Energy is directed to one part of the body and is held there with attention for a specified length of time to increase the power of that particular area. In this way, the *mudras* contribute to the systematic awakening of the *kundalini shakti* (the cosmic force inherent in all individuals). With the exception of *viparita karani mudra* (the headstand), the *mudras* are all executed in seated positions.

In a *mudra,* the combination of controlled posture, regulated respiration with breath retention, and *bandhas* is used to hold this power and the mind within a center in the subtle body. The energy of that center is then drawn up into the center above it, and this process is repeated all the way to the crown chakra. In this way, a *mudra* is a process, through which obstructions in the subtle channels are removed and the power of the subtle body is strengthened and refined. At the same time, on another level, the attachments and rigid patterns of the mind are dissolved. The *Hatha Pradipika* of Svatmarama, the most authoritative text on hatha yoga, describes ten *mudras;* the *Gheranda Samhita* lists twenty-five; and the *Yoga Pradipika* of Jayatarama speaks of twenty-four sealing processes.

The ten *mudras* mentioned by Svatmarama are *mahamudra, mahabandha, maha vedha, khechari, uddiyana, mulabandha, jalandhara bandha, viparita karani, vajroli,* and *shakti chalana.* Most of these *mudras* do not need to be practiced by all, since they are intended for the removal of specific energetic obstructions. The exceptions are *uddiyana, mulabandha* and *jalandhara, khechari, viparita karani,* and *shakti chalana mudras.* These should be used at all times for the concentration and the elevation of the *kundalini shakti. Mahamudra* helps in overcoming energetic blockages in the three lower chakras. These three chakras (*muladhara, swadhisthana,* and *manipura*) are in charge of respiration, heat, and stability. Together these produce the increase in power. When there is a buildup of fluid or over-growth of muscle between the perineal center and the diaphragm, *mahamudra* is used for the reduction of these excesses. This frees the pranic force from domination by greed-infected activities like eating, drinking, sex, or overactivity of any kind.

Mahabandha is the combination of *uddiyana, mulabandha,* and *jalandhara* and helps to overcome blockages in the heart and throat centers, including blockages arising from mental imposition. *Maha vedha* is a development of *mahabandha* that helps to shake the pranic force free from the base chakra and then pierce through, all the way to the crown chakra.

There are individuals who can clear the inner pathways through the practices of asana, *kriya,* and *pranayama* alone (with the application of the three *bandhas*). For such people these three *mudras* are not required.

The three *bandhas* are the true kings of the hermetic isolation of the pranic force. Without them, none of the *mudras* would be effective.

Khechari mudra training should only be started with the advice of, and under the guidance of, an experienced teacher. *Viparita karani mudra (sirsasana)* has two functions. It reduces the number of respirations per minute and eventually it can lead to a complete stoppage of respiration. By this practice, the movement of breath, the heartbeat, and the fluctuations of the mind are brought under voluntary control. In addition, *viparita karani mudra* also cultivates *pratyahara* (sense withdrawal), which is the link between the external *(bahiranga)* and the internal *(antaranga)* practices. *Pratyahara* is achieved through a number of different techniques. The best of these to practice initially is given in the *Vasishta Samhita* and the *Gorakshashatakam*. These texts recommend holding *viparita karani mudra* while systematically concentrating the pranic force and then moving it through a chain of sixteen (some schools say eighteen) vital points. To be able to practice in this way *sirsasana* must be mastered first.

According to Sri T. Krishnamacharya, the practice of asana, *kriya, bandha, pranayama,* and *mudra* is enough until the age of sixty. The practice of *pratyahara* should only begin at this stage of life. This advice intimates that the correct practice of yoga should be in harmony with the unfolding of the energies of life. If things are forced before their time, violation occurs, and this will result in injury or terminal disease. In such ways are efforts wasted because of impatience, fear, greed, and lack of wisdom.

Shakti chalana mudra (churning of the power) is the combination of *bhastrika* and *suryabhedana pranayamas* with the performance of *nauli kriya* during *bhaya kumbhaka*. The time allotted for this practice is from one to two and a half hours. The practice of all the *mudras* should be learned under the supervision of an experienced teacher. Until such a teacher is available, they should be left alone.

The terms *vajroli, amaroli,* and *sahajoli* describe essentially the same process. The names differ, but their functions are the same. These practices are elaborately explained in most of the hatha yoga texts. In the *Yukta Bhavadeva,* Bhavadeva Mishra suggests that these three practices are only prescribed for perversely infatuated and ignorant people. It may be added that there are much better ways to facilitate the upward movement of semen and ova. Sexual energy cannot be controlled through suppression and denial. Such control evolves naturally out of a growing understanding of the energetic principles of the yogic practices.

14
Laya (Absorption)

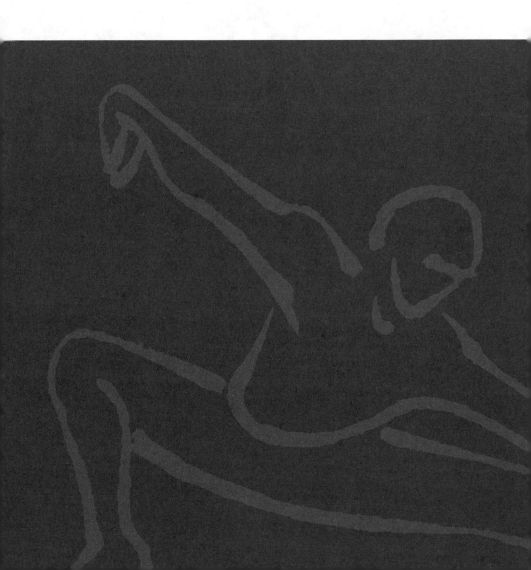

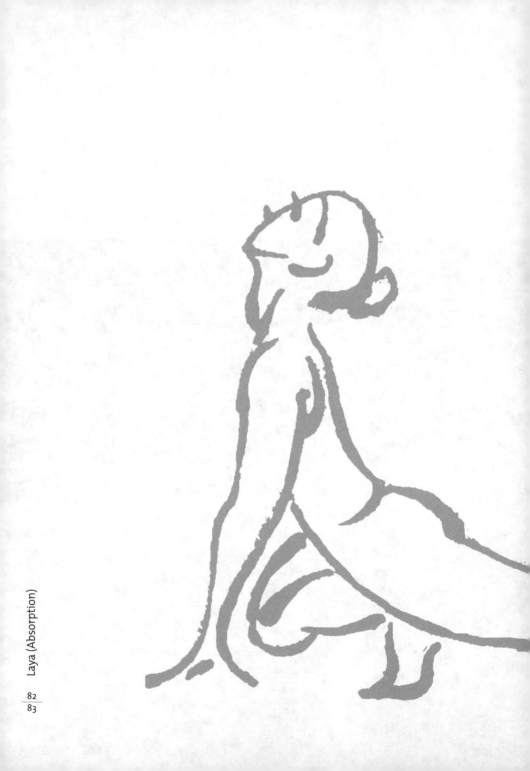

Laya is the process of absorption achieved in hatha yoga through the practice of *nadanusandana* (listening to the inner sound). It corresponds to the practice of *samyama* described in the *Yoga Sutras* of Patanjali, which consists of the three stages *dharana* (concentration), *dhyana* (meditation), and *samadhi* (which also means absorption).

All these practices of *antaranga sadhana* require an advanced refinement of the mind. This is the true goal of the *bahiranga sadhana,* and if these earlier stages are not mastered there is no way forward, however ardent or committed the practitioner may be.

The energetic cultivation achieved through the stages of asana, *kriya, bandha, pranayama, mudra,* and *pratyahara* creates an unobstructed field of energy in which the internal and external forces dissolve into each other. These forces then act as one unified power. This final point of the *bahiranga sadhana* is the starting point for the *antaranga* and *paramantaranga sadhanas,* which are the goal of all the yogas.

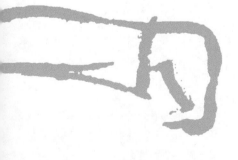

Part 2
Application

1
Preludes
(Diagrams)

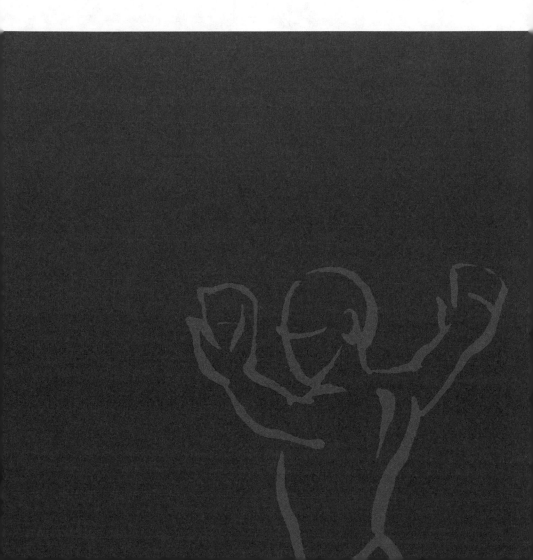

Balakrama (Stepping into Strength)

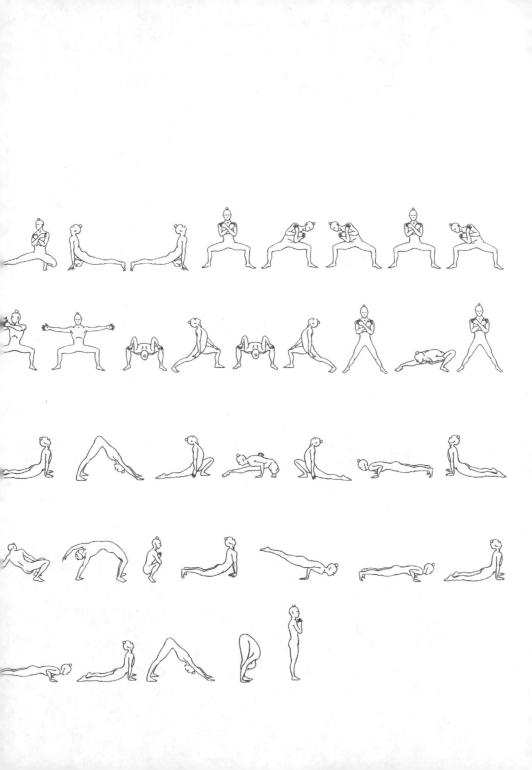

Chaya Yoddha Sancalanam
(Churning of the Shadow Warrior)

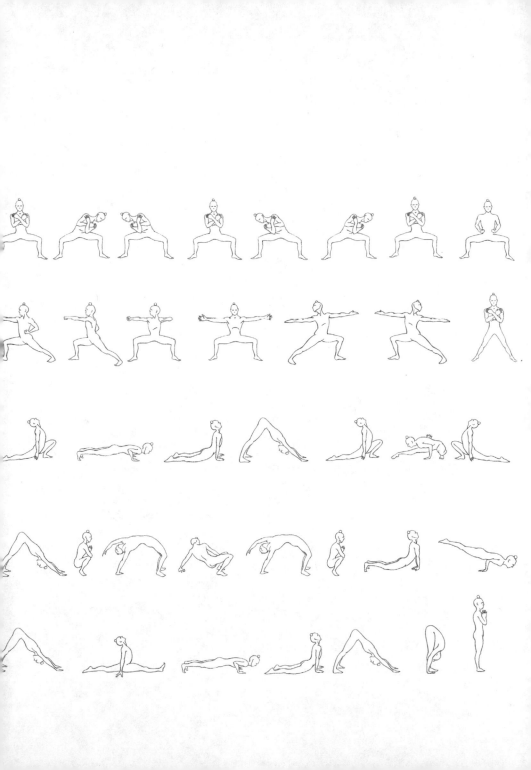

Karttikeya Mandala
(Garland of Light)

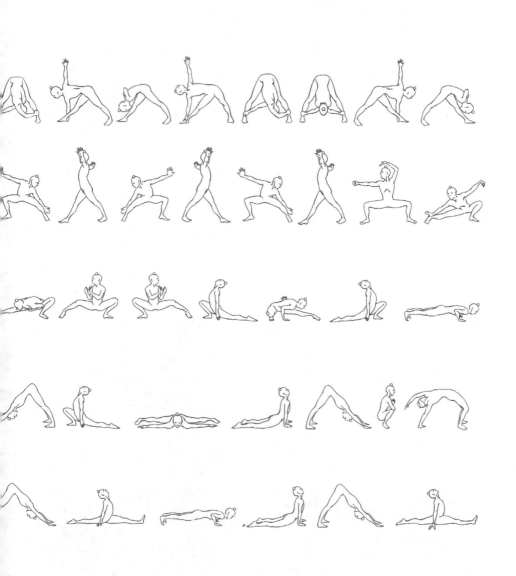

2
Asanas (Photos)

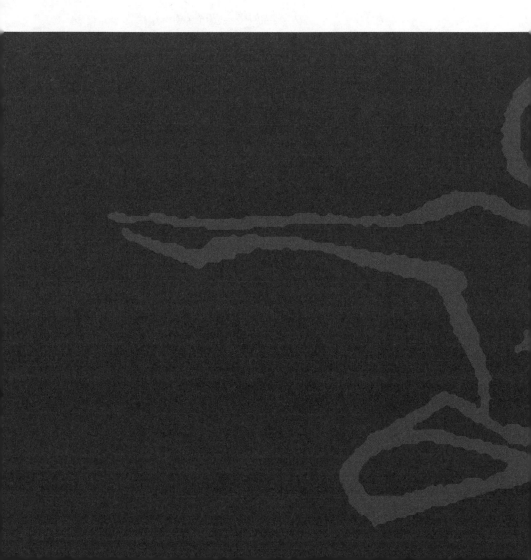

Asana

Asana (seat) should be firm, light and at ease through the control of the body's natural tendencies by meditation on the infinite.

Patanjali, Yoga Sutras II, 47

The effort for the achievement is done only for the maintenance of the body's life. It is not a tool for asana. By being the accidental case for asana, it may ruin the laws of asana.

Vyasabhasya

One should arrive at an asana through adaptation and not by imposition, as Patanjali's sutra and Vyasa's comment on it clearly state. This can only be achieved by choosing the simplest of asanas in order to awaken the vivid state of alertness.

The process for the seats should be via the coded patterns of the prelude forms that are designed for overcoming energetic obstructions of the body, rendering the mind sensitive toward the action. In selecting asanas to reveal the practical side of this book's intellectual content, the most uncomplicated and simplest were chosen.

To ensure a smooth and positive transition, these asanas should be learned slowly, with patience, and under an experienced guide.

1. Baddha Konasana

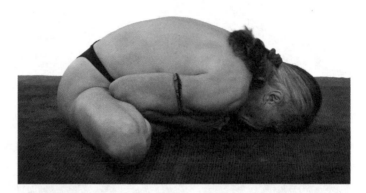

Baddha Konasana (bound angle pose) directly tones the liver, spleen, and stomach while indirectly influencing the heart and the pancreas.

2. Gorakshasana

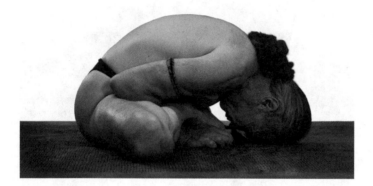

Gorakshasana is named after the great hatha yoga master Gorakshanatha. This pose tones the kidneys, relaxes the heart, and stimulates the muladhara chakra.

3. Mulabandasana

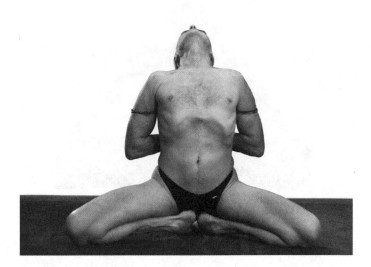

Mulabandasana (the root posture) strengthens the perineal regions and the root of the bladder including the eight divisions of the lower limbs—hips, knees, ankles, and feet.

4. Mandukasana

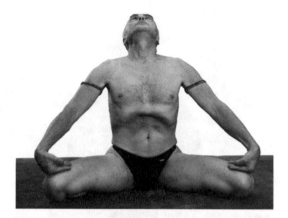

Mandukasana (seat of the frog) removes stiffness of the upper and lower limbs and promotes the spontaneous retention of the breath.

5. Kurmasana

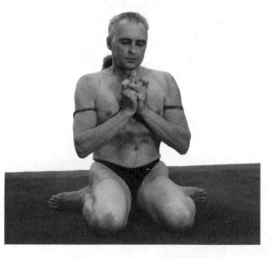

Kurmasana (seat of the tortoise) purifies the entire body of the eighty-four diseases inflicted by wind (vata), thus causing softness and stability within the body's joints.

6. *Vamadevasana*

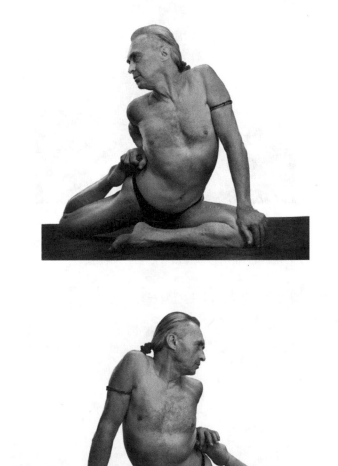

Vamadevasana is named after one of Lord Shiva's incarnations. This pose eases the hardness of the sacral and groin regions, preparing the spine for backward bending.

7. Padmasana

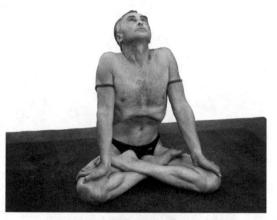

Padmasana (the lotus seat), besides being the most popular seat for the practices of pranayama and meditation, also heals ailments of the body and cures diseases.

8. Baddha Padmasana

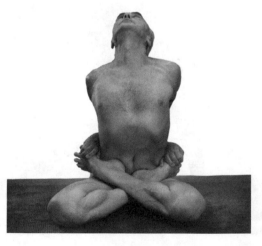

Baddha Padmasana (the bound lotus seat), in addition to the uses and benefits mentioned under padmasana, is intended for advanced-level students of pranayama.

Glossary

Adharas: vital supports

Adhipati: crown of the head

Agni: inner fire

Ahimsa: nonviolence

Ajna chakra: subtle energy center at the third eye

Alambusha: one of the thirteen main nadis that transport prana around the body

Amantrakam: the use of numbers to count the breath

Anahata chakra: subtle energy at the heart

Anandamaya kosha: trap of joy

Annamaya kosha: trap of food

Antara kumbhaka: retention of breath following an inhalation

Antaranga sadhana: internal practices of yoga, meditative states

Antaryami: the indwelling soul

Anuloma: with the hair

Apanavayu: downward moving wind of the body, elimination

Ardha chandrasana: half-moon pose, standing

Arohan: upward channel of sushumna

Asana: seat, pose

Ashtanga: eight limbs

Atha: then, now

Atma: the supreme soul

Avadhuta yoga: asceticism, the skillful use of the equipment of hatha yoga

Avarohan: downward channel of sushumna

Avritti: dissipating motion

Ayama: a lengthening process, as in pranayama

Baddha padmasana: bound lotus

Bahiranga sadhana: external practices of yoga, asana, kriya, bandha, pranayama, mudra, pratyahara

Bandha: lock, tie

Bhadrasana: friendly pose

Bharatanatya: style of dance from southern India

Bhastri, also *bhastrika:* the bellows breath, a type of pranayama

Bhaya kumbhaka, also *bahir kumbhaka:* retention of breath following an exhalation

Bhekasana: frog pose

Bhujangasana: cobra pose

Bramhari: the humming breath, a type of pranayama

Chakra: subtle inner energy center

Chalani: see nauli kriya

Chaya: shadow

Chaya vivaranam: opening the shadow

Chaya Yoddha Sancalanam: churning of the shadow warrior

Dharana: concentration

Dhatu: tissue

Dhyana: meditation

Dosha: constitution or humor

Gandhari: one of the thirteen main nadis that transport prana around the body

Ghati: twenty-four minutes, unit of time

Hastijiva: one of the thirteen main nadis that transport prana around the body

Hatha: ha = sun, *tha* = moon, merging of opposite energies

Hrdayam: the heart space

Ida nadi: the left nostril, the lunar channel

Indriya: sense organ

Jalandhara: one of the three main bandhas and one of the ten main mudras

Janu sirsasana: a seated forward bend

Jiva: individual soul

Jiva bandha: lock of the soul, a type of bandha

Jivatman, also *antaryami:* the indwelling soul

Jnanendriyas: five senses related to perception organs

Kaivalya: isolation

Kalaripayyat: an Indian style of martial arts

Kanda: pot or bulb, situated below the manipura chakra

Kandara: sinews

Kapalabhati: shining of the skull, a type of pranayama

Kapha: one of the three main Ayurvedic doshas, earth/water

Karana sharira: the causal body

Karmendriyas: organs of action (mouth, hands, feet, genitals, anus)

Kathakali: style of dance from southern India

Kaya: the body

Ketu: the south node of the moon

Kevala kumbhaka: spontaneous cessation of the breath

Khechari: one of the ten main mudras

Kosha: entrapment, trap, sheath

Kriya: process

Kuhu: one of the thirteen main nadis that transport prana around the body

Kukkutasana: rooster pose

Kumbhaka: retention of breath

Kundalini shakti: the cosmic force inherent in individuals

Kurmasana: tortoise pose

Lahari: the floating breath, a type of pranayama

Lauliki: see nauli kriya

Laya, also *samadhi:* absorption

Maha: great

Maha vedha: one of the ten main mudras

Maha yoga: great yoga

Mahabandha: a combination of jalandhara, mulabandha, and uddiyana; one of the ten main mudras

Mahamudra: one of the ten main mudras

Manas: the thinking, processing mind

Mandukasana: seated frog pose

Manipura chakra: inner energy center at the solar plexus

Manomaya kosha: the trap of the processing mind

Marma: a junction or point of subtle energy

Marmasthana: the science of marmas

Mayurasana: peacock pose

Mitahara: controlled intake of pure food

Mrigi mudra: gesture of the deer

Mudra: gesture

Mukha: face

Mulabandha: one of the three main bandhas and one of the ten main mudras

Muladhara chakra: a subtle energy center at the base of the spine

Murcha: the swooning breath, a type of pranayama

Nadanusandana: the unstruck sound

Nadi: subtle energy channel

Nadi granthi: knots within the central channel of sushumna

Nadi shodhana: cleansing of the channels, a type of pranayama

Nagadi vayus: sub-winds situated in and around the heart

Nauli kriya: churning of the abdominal wall to purify the digestive tract

Nauliki: see nauli kriya

Niyamas: observances regarding one's behavior

Omkara: gesture of om, a mudra

Pancha: five

Pancha karma: the five cleansing acts used in Ayurveda

Paramantaranga sadhana: the supreme practice

Paramatma: supreme soul

Parivritti: spiraling

Paschimottanasana: seated forward bend

Pasha: noose or reins

Pashu: animalistic existence

Pashupati: the shining herdsman

Pati: mastery

Phana: hood, a marma point on the nose that affects breathing

Pingala nadi: channel of the right nostril, the solar channel

Pitta: one of the three main Ayurvedic doshas, fire/water

Plavini: see lahari

Prana: life force

Pranamaya kosha: the trap of power

Pranasamyama: even restraint of the life force

Pranavayu: the central wind located in the heart

Pranayama: practices of lengthening the breath

Pratiloma: combination of anuloma and viloma

Pratyahara: withdrawal from the sensory world

Puraka: inhalation

Pusha: one of the thirteen main nadis that transport prana around the body

Rahu: the north node of the moon

Raja yoga: royal yoga

Rechaka: exhalation

Sadhaka: student, one with a spiritual practice

Sadhaka pitta: internal fire, heat that builds during practice

Sadhana: spiritual practice

Sahasrara chakra: subtle energy center at the crown of the head

Sahita kumbhaka: imposed cessation of the breath

Sama: same, equal

Samadhi: absorption

Samanavayu: equalizing wind, seated in the navel; assimilation

Samantrakam: the use of a mantra to count the breath

Samavritti: even rhythm, an even ratio of inhale and exhale

Samyama: even restraint

Saraswati nadi: channel of the tongue

Shakti: cosmic energy

Shakti chalana: one of the ten main mudras

Shakti chalana mudra: the churning or raising of power

Shankini: one of the thirteen main nadis that transport prana around the body

Shatkarma: the six cleansing processes

Shitali: a cooling breath, a type of pranayama

Shivani: fibrous sutures

Shrotas: channels

Siddha: attained; a sage, a seer

Siddhasana: adept pose

Sirsasana, also *viparita karani mudra:* headstand

Sitkari: a cooling breath, a type of pranayama

Smashana: burning grounds

Sthana: bodily stance

Sthula sharira: the gross body

Sukshma sharira: the subtle body

Suryabhedana: piercing the sun, a type of pranayama

Sushumna nadi: fire channel

Swadhisthana chakra: an inner energy center below the solar plexus

Swastikasana: sun wheel

Tantra: system of philosophy

Tantrika: practitioner of tantra

Tantrikam: see amantrakam

Udanavayu: upward moving wind, seated at the throat

Uddiyana: one of the three main bandhas and one of the ten main mudras

Ujjayi: the victorious breath, a type of pranayama

Urdhva dhanurasana: back bend

Vajrini nadi: thrusting channel

Vajroli: one of the ten main mudras

Varuni: one of the thirteen main nadis that transport prana around the body

Vasishta: Vedic seer

Vata: one of the three main Ayurvedic doshas, ether/air

Vayu: wind force of prana moving within the body

Vijnanamaya kosha: trap of the intuitive intellect

Viloma: against the hair

Vinyasa: placement

Viparita karani mudra: one of the ten main mudras, the headstand

Vishamavritti: an uneven ratio of inhale and exhale

Vishvodhara: one of the thirteen main nadis that transport prana around the body

Vishuddha chakra: subtle energy center at the throat

Vyanavayu: circulating wind, seated in the skin

Yamas: restraints regarding one's behavior

Yashashvini: one of the thirteen main nadis that transport prana around the body

Yoganga sadhana: yogic practices

Yonisthana: perineal floor

Bibliography

Danielou, Alain, trans. *La Siva Svarodaya*. Milan: Arche, 1982.

Gharote, M., and V. A. Bedekar, trans. *Yogayajnavalkya Samhita*. Pune, India: Kaivalyadhama S.M.Y.M. Samiti, 1982.

Gorakshanatha. *Gorakshashatakam*. Translated by Swami Kuvalayananda and S. A. Samiti. Pune, India: Kaivalyadhama S.M.Y.M. Samiti, n.d.

———. *Siddha Siddhanta Padati*. Translated by M. Gharote. Pune, India: Lonavla Yoga Institute, 2005.

Kaivalyadhama Institute, trans. *Vasishta Samhita*. Pune, India: Kaivalyadhama S.M.Y.M. Samiti, 1984.

Krishnamacharya, Sri T. *Salutations to the Teacher and the Eternal One*. Unpublished manuscript from transcribed talks of Krishnamacharya.

Krishnamacharya, Sri T. *Yogasana*. [In Kannada.] India, n.d.

Mishra, Bhavadeva. *Yukta Bhavadeva*. Translated by M. Gharote. Pune, India: Lonavla Yoga Institute, 2002.

Patanjali. *Yoga Sutras*. Translated by Bangali Baba. Delhi: Motilal Banarsidass, 1975.

Srinivasa, Yogi. *Hatha Ratnavali*. Translated by M. Gharote. Pune, India: Lonavla Yoga Institute, 2004.

Svatmarama. *Hatha Yoga Pradipika*. Translated by Jyotsna of Brahmananda. Chennai, India: Adyar Library & Research Center, 1972.

Vasu, Rai Bahadur Sris Chandra, trans. *Siva Samhita*. Delhi: Munshiram Manoharlal, 1975.

Vasu, Sris Chandra, trans. *Gheranda Samhita*. Adyar, India: Theosophical Publishing House, 1895.

Zvelebil, Kamil V. *The Poets of the Powers*. London: Rider & Co., 1973.

———. *The Siddha Quest for Immortality*. Oxford: Mandrake of Oxford, 1996.